MATRIX
HEALING

Discover Your Greatest Health Potential
Through the Power of Kabbalah

MATRIX
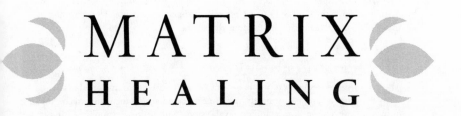
HEALING

RAPHAEL KELLMAN, M.D.
Foreword by Larry Dossey, M.D.

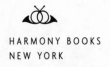

HARMONY BOOKS
NEW YORK

Grateful acknowledgment is made to the following for permission to reprint previously published material:

ArtScroll/Mesorah Publications: Stories adapted from *Not Just Stories* by Rabbi Abraham J. Twerski, M.D. Adapted by permission of Shaar Press; ArtScroll/Mesorah Publications.

Crown Publishers: Stories adapted from *A Treasury of Jewish Folklore* by Nathan Ausubel. Copyright © 1948, 1976 by Crown Publishers, Inc. Adapted by permission of Crown Publishers, a division of Random House, Inc.

Published by Harmony Books, New York, New York. Member of the Crown Publishing Group, a division of Random House, Inc.
www.crownpublishing.com

HARMONY BOOKS is a registered trademark and the Harmony Books colophon is a trademark of Random House, Inc.

Printed in the United States of America

Design by Elina D. Nudelman

Library of Congress Cataloging-in-Publication Data

Kellman, Raphael, 1960–
    Matrix healing : discover your greatest health potential through the power of Kabbalah / Raphael Kellman.— 1st ed.
    1. Kabbalah—Health aspects. 2. Spiritual healing and spiritualism. 3. Health—Religious aspects—Judaism. 4. Mysticism—Health aspects. I. Title.
    RZ999K45 2004
    615.8'52—dc22

                                                                    2004001694

ISBN 1-4000-4896-6

10 9 8 7 6 5 4 3 2 1

First Edition

To my niece Jordana, who came into this world too small to conceal the beauty of her soul, and who evoked within us a wellspring of love and compassion. Her life is already a Blessing.

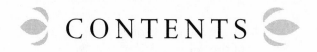

CONTENTS

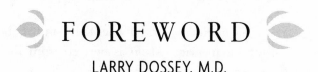

FOREWORD

LARRY DOSSEY, M.D.

MATRIX HEALING involves a journey that has been trailblazed in the past by countless individuals often referred to as mystics—individuals who have an inner drive to comprehend reality fully and personally, unmediated by any institution or authority. Their ultimate goal is utterly audacious—to unite with the Divine—and their legacy is the accumulated wisdom of some of the greatest seers and visionaries in history.

The urge toward mystical understanding is universal; we know of no cultures where mystical traditions do not occur. And although there are profound cultural and religious differences in how mystical understanding is expressed, an underlying thread connects all the various mystical paths—thus, the saying that all mystics come from the same country and speak the same language.

Matrix Healing presents readers with life-changing lessons and practical guidelines that can heal, but it is the profundity and power of the eternal mystical vision, expressed through the Jewish tradition of Kabbalah, that constitutes the real juice of this book and distinguishes it from self-help, how-to books on healing.

Matrix Healing: Dr. Raphael Kellman has chosen a perfect title for his message. *Matrix* is derived from the Latin *mater,* from whence comes *mother,* and refers to "womb," "source," and "origin." *Matrix* is, therefore, a splendid referent to mysticism, which is the search for the source of all there is. And *healing,* which is derived from the Anglo-Saxon *helan,* "to make whole," expresses the same sentiment.

Why link mystical and spiritual traditions with healing, as Dr. Kellman has courageously done? Throughout history they have usually been united, and many of humankind's greatest spiritual teachers were gifted healers. History is peppered with instances in which people who suffered from terrible diseases were healed following revelations and epiphanies, or who ventured into the orbit of spiritual masters and emerged whole. Unfortunately, in modern medicine we have largely forgotten this connection. As a result, we have consigned spirituality to the province of formal religion and, having equated healing with curing, have relegated it to medical science.

We have paid a high price for this division of labor. We have come to believe that illness and disease are completely physical in origin, solely the result of malfunctioning atoms, molecules, and organs, with no influence from mind, consciousness, or spirit. During the twentieth century, believing otherwise became scientifically incorrect, a sign of intellectual softheadedness. Not only did the concept of spirit disappear from medical science, the notions of mind and consciousness also became endangered. For example, entire textbooks of neurology were written during the past century in which the concept of mind completely disappeared.

Fortunately, we are in the process of regaining our balance in these matters. In the past two decades, an increasing number of studies have documented the crucial interplay of body, mind, and spirit. Currently, more than 1,200 studies suggest that if people follow a spiritual path in their life—it does not appear to matter which—they experience on average a lower incidence of all major diseases and live significantly longer than people who do not follow such a path. In addition, several studies suggest that prayer and compassionate intentions can evoke healing responses in distant individuals, even when those individuals are unaware that such efforts are being made on their behalf. These studies have generated immense interest, but also controversy, because they call into question the conventional assumptions about the nature of consciousness and how it manifests in the world. On balance, these findings suggest that we have underestimated the healing power of the mind and that our predecessors, who believed in an intimate connection between spirituality and healing, were correct.

In the pages that follow, Dr. Kellman lays out specific techniques and instructions designed to help anyone achieve greater health. Some theologically minded individuals may be concerned that this emphasis on practicality may dishonor the mystical and spiritual side of life. If spiritual methods are used to promote health, spirituality may come to be regarded in purely pragmatic or utilitarian terms, as just another tool in the physician's black bag. It is true that people incessantly use spiritual practices for the most mundane reasons, such as praying to win the lottery or to find a parking space. But although spiritual practices *can* be demeaned by an excessive practical emphasis, that does not mean that the commonplace needs of daily life should be off-limits to spiritual interventions. After all, Jesus urged his followers to pray for their daily bread, which for a hungry person is practical, indeed.

I greatly admire Dr. Kellman, a fellow internist, for writing *Matrix Healing* and reminding us that we are composite creatures made up of body, mind, and spirit. Physicians all over the country are rediscovering this ancient awareness, and I am amazed by how creatively they often integrate this understanding into their practice. As an example, a physician friend of mine, who became impressed with the experimental evidence favoring the healing power of prayer, decided that he should utilize prayer in his practice of internal medicine. How, he wondered, could he do this sensitively, without intruding into his patients' personal lives? He settled on a simple solution: a three-sentence printed statement, which his receptionist gave to each patient who entered his office. It said, "I have reviewed the scientific evidence surrounding prayer, and I believe prayer might help you. As your physician, I choose to pray for you. However, if you do not wish me to do so, simply sign this statement below and return it to my receptionist, and I will not add you to my prayer list." Over several years, the number of patients who signed and returned the sheet, declining his prayers, was *zero.* This incident indicates not just that physicians are willing to go in the directions Dr. Kellman proposes, but that most patients are actually hungry for them to do so.

Those who fear that scientific medicine will be compromised by spiritually based approaches need not worry. We have entered an era in which it is becoming unscientific *not* to address spiritual concerns in medical care. Many physicians realize this and are delighted by this turnaround. One reason physicians feel this way is that they have spiritual needs just like anyone else, and it is not fulfilling to practice medicine as if patients are little more than skin-encapsulated bags of meat.

The methods and techniques of *Matrix Healing* do not require anyone to give up conventional approaches such as drugs and surgical procedures. Scientific medicine will not only survive an infusion of spirituality, it will be enhanced and rejuvenated. Dr. Kellman keenly realizes this. He is an internist who has paid his dues and is at home in modern medicine. He knows that a healing method that emphasizes only one side, whether the physical or the spiritual, is unbalanced. His is a complementary, integrated approach, not an either/or method.

Matrix Healing is the clearest explanation of Kabbalah healing principles I have seen. Dr. Kellman has captured the power and wisdom of this great tradition, which he shares without trivializing. This book's message transcends specific religious traditions because all authentic wisdom is ultimately universal. That is why *Matrix Healing* can be a unifying force between all cultures and traditions—and what could be more important in our troubled times?

Matrix: mother, source, origin. *Healing:* wholeness, oneness. These words convey comfort, consolation, and completeness. May *Matrix Healing* help you find this awareness and the realization that, in some dimension, you are already perfect as you are.

—LARRY DOSSEY, M.D.,
author of *Healing Beyond the Body,*
Reinventing Medicine, and *Healing Words*

I have seen that all those sparks flash from the High Spark . . . .
All those lights are connected:
this light to that light, that light to this light,
one shining into the other,
inseparable one from the other.

—THE ZOHAR

I shall give you a new heart, and I shall put a new spirit within
you. I shall remove the heart of stone from within you, and give
you a heart of flesh.

—EZEKIEL 36:26

MATRIX
HEALING

INTRODUCTION: 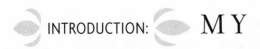 MY JOURNEY TO MATRIX HEALING

JOSÉ ORTEGA Y GASSET–

> *To be surprised, to wonder, is to begin to understand.*

WHEN I think about my journey to Matrix Healing, I realize that it started in childhood. I was the kind of child who just couldn't stop wondering about the world. "Why is the sky blue? How come I can talk and a dog can't? Why do we say a prayer before we eat?— who's listening, and why do they care?" As I grew older, the questions grew more complex, but I never stopped wondering.

At first, I thought that religion might have the answers I sought. I was brought up in an Orthodox Jewish household, so my religious education began quite early. But to my frustration, the religious school I attended provided me with only a small portion of the knowledge I sought. Though I couldn't have put my feelings into words, I somehow sensed that something was missing.

Now, don't get me wrong. I was proud of being Jewish, and I enjoyed learning about Jewish laws and traditions. I looked forward to the many Jewish holidays we celebrated, each with its own rituals, its special foods and ceremonies. But I wanted a sense of the bigger picture, an understanding of how I could access the divine in my own life. Religious education did a wonderful job of sharing facts and history—but my soul was craving more.

As a result, I lost interest pretty quickly in the conventional way of understanding Judaism. It wasn't a case of agreeing or disagreeing. I simply sensed a hunger inside me that wasn't being fed.

As a young man, I thought maybe this hunger could be satisfied by a different religion. I studied Buddhism, Hinduism, and Sufism, wondering if these traditions would illuminate life's mysteries for me. At the same time, I also studied science. Perhaps, I reasoned, the men and women who probed the atom or explored the farthest reaches of space were the ones who could tell me what life was really made of.

Of course, it wasn't simply theoretical knowledge I was seeking. I wanted a way to improve my own life. Wisdom, I thought, meant understanding life so well that you could savor it to the fullest. Wisdom would expand my capacity for joy and fulfillment, enabling me to access both the sensual and the spiritual joys of life.

Yet, despite my studies of science, philosophy, and religion, I found nothing that felt remotely like the wisdom I was looking for. It disturbed me that science appeared so sure of itself when virtually all scientific discoveries seemed eventually doomed to obsolescence. After all, top scientists had once believed that the sun revolved around the earth, and that Newton's Second Law of Thermodynamics was the last word in physics. Then Copernicus, Galileo, and Einstein came along, followed by other scientists who superseded *them*. How could today's scientists be so arrogant, knowing that their own theories would soon be out-of-date?

Religion, as I then understood it, seemed equally unsatisfying. I longed for a world infused with the presence of the divine, a world that was not about serving some faraway deity but rather about discovering the God within ourselves. But whether the fault was in my professors, myself, or both, the religions I studied did not seem to speak to this need.

Eventually, an interest in healing led me to medical school. Perhaps, I thought, when I saw the healing role science played in people's lives, I would begin to grasp its spiritual aspect and bring science and religion together.

No such luck. For one thing, I soon realized that the science that formed the basis for modern Western medicine was sadly outdated. The anatomy, physiology, and other subjects taught in U.S. medical schools are based on a mechanistic approach to the human body that dates back to the seventeenth century, with particular influence from the views of eighteenth-century French philosopher René Descartes. Descartes saw the universe as a gigantic machine, with us humans as tiny cogs within it. In this mechanistic world, our minds and souls were completely separate from our physical selves—irrelevant to understanding the body. This was the worldview that dominated—and still dominates—virtually every U.S. medical school.

Today, I can cite numerous studies showing that even from a purely scientific point of view, this mechanistic approach is sadly outdated. Much of this book is devoted to explaining how, and to putting forth an alternative that, back then, I could sense only dimly: that we humans are composed of body, mind, soul, and spirit. All the different systems of our body work together to form a whole that is somehow greater than the sum of our parts. Each of us is part of a larger whole, as well, so that if any one of us is sick—or if our planet is—then all of us need healing.

Needless to say, I found little support for this holistic, spiritual perspective in medical school! Moreover, the mechanistic view of science seemed to lead to a kind of arrogance and coldness that I found profoundly disturbing. I remember one day on rounds, a group of residents were gathered around a young man who had gone into a coma. As I glanced down at our patient's smooth young face and jet-black hair, I felt a deep sorrow at the thought of this brief life that had suddenly been cut so short. Tests had revealed that he had virtually no brain activity. Clearly, he was doomed to die.

I looked around at my colleagues. Surely they shared my grief at this loss of human potential. After all, most of us were barely older than this man ourselves.

Yet as I listened to the conversation around me, I realized that the only thing of interest to this group of intelligent, sophisticated people was the reflex test they were discussing—a procedure in which a doctor put water in the young man's ear and then reviewed his responses. Suddenly, I felt sick to my stomach and abruptly walked off the floor.

The next time I saw the attending physician, he asked me why I'd left. "Well," I said slowly, "it was what we were talking about. There was so much more going on than just a reflex test. . . ."

"What did you say?" he replied in a confused way. Although I was speaking in a normal tone of voice, what I was saying was so far outside his frame of reference that he literally couldn't hear me.

"It's not important," I said. "I just needed some fresh air." I looked at him again. He was a kind and sensitive man, known for his unusual patience and generosity with both his students and his patients. Most doctors in his position would probably not even have bothered to ask me if anything was wrong. It wasn't a personal failing of his that I was responding to, but a failure in the framework he was part of. What was missing seemed so basic, so fundamental. With all our technology, drugs, and intelligence, we would never be able to create real health in our patients—because we were lacking compassion.

I recall another set of rounds, this time led by the respected head of our intensive care unit. This man was extremely bright, well respected, prominent in the community and in our hospital. He was also known as a religious person—but, of course, while we were on rounds, not a word was spoken about spiritual matters or the role of the mind in healing. Instead, the talk was all of wonder drugs, cardiac output, hemodynamic status, vascular resistance. You could feel the sense of pride that every one of us shared as this eminent physician rattled off the technical terms, explaining the latest advances in cardiology that enabled us to save more lives than ever before.

One day I saw this doctor praying, and I was bewildered. He had all of this incredible knowledge, yet he was bowing his head to God, as though the realm of science had abruptly ended and God had simply taken over. Not that I was opposed to prayer—on the contrary—but I wondered why this doctor couldn't integrate the roles that the mind, soul, and consciousness played in healing. Why couldn't his science include a sense of mystery and wonder, even as his religion empowered him to intervene effectively in the world? Weren't there spiritual and metaphysical laws that we humans might follow to affect the physical world? Once again, I was struck by the apparently unbridgeable gap between the arrogance of science and the helplessness of religion. Wasn't there any way to bring the two together?

These questions continued to plague me throughout my residency and on into my first few years of practice as a physician. Although I explored holistic medicine and always tried to treat my patients in an integrated, respectful way, I felt increasingly distressed by the gap between the spiritual hunger I sensed in my patients and the technological medicine I was able to offer them.

Then I discovered Kabbalah.

ENCOUNTERING KABBALAH

> I never imagined when I began my career as a physicist that I would one day be writing *qua* physicist that Heaven exists and that we shall each and every one of us enjoy life after death. But here I am writing what my younger self would regard as scientific nonsense. Here I stand, as a physicist, I can do no other.
>
> —FRANK J. TIPLER

When I recently read that quote from Frank J. Tipler, I was struck by a sense of irony. Tipler, a physicist, was shocked that his beloved science had demonstrated—almost against his will—the existence of God, the importance of the soul, even the possibility of resurrection. Today he is known for his pioneering work in integrating physics, computer science—and theology.

I, on the other hand, had started my journey with a kind of soul hunger that I had begun to doubt science could ever fulfill. Only when I encountered Kabbalah did I discover the marriage of science and religion that I had been seeking all my life. Finally, the physical and spiritual dimensions began to merge into a new world.

From an early age, I had been vaguely aware of Kabbalah as a mystical tradition within Judaism. All I really knew was that it was supposed to be a kind of secret knowledge, and that my rabbi considered it basically irrelevant to the practice of the Jewish religion.

As I was finishing my residency, I came upon some books about Kabbalah that for some reason caught my eye. Although I had previously thought of Kabbalah as springing out of Judaism, I began to realize that, instead, Judaism is rooted in Kabbalah. In fact, Kabbalah is no more of a religion than quantum physics is. Rather, Kabbalah's main spiritual underpinnings offer a new worldview for all human beings, no matter what their religion or even if they have rejected all religion. Kabbalah, I learned, is a spiritual perspective that had always been intended for the entire human race.

The founding text of Kabbalah is the Zohar, a 2,000-year-old book based on an oral tradition that had existed for thousands of years. For most of that time, the tradition had been cloaked in a secrecy considered necessary because the vision put forth in the Zohar was so advanced that, until our own time, almost no one would have been able to understand it. If you read the Zohar with modern eyes, you realize that the early kabbalists knew about electricity. They knew the earth was round, with a North Pole and a South Pole. They even knew that the earth revolved around the sun—centuries before Copernicus! Indeed, much of their vision was remarkably close to that of the quantum physicists who revolutionized scientific thought in the early twentieth century. How could such advanced knowledge have been made widely available during the first two millennia? The world was hardly ready for this radical new way of thinking.

In the late twentieth and early twenty-first centuries, however, popular understanding has finally caught up with the insights of the kabbalists, even as modern physics has prepared us to understand their way of thinking. By now we have grown as human beings, with a more sophisticated and spiritual worldview and true insight into our role and power in the world.

THE PROMISE OF KABBALAH

Thou hast made known unto me thy deep mysterious things.

—THE BOOK OF HYMNS, THE DEAD SEA SCROLLS

My study of Kabbalah took me on an extraordinary journey in which the insights of quantum physics gained a whole new meaning. Although our senses show us just one universe— a universe that contains pain, suffering, disease, and death— Kabbalah explains that there exists not just one universe, but many. Side by side exist an infinite number of parallel universes with multiple possibilities. Once we know of their existence, we can choose to access them, including the universe in which we are all already healed, happy, and perfectly fulfilled, the universe in which we are perfectly united with one another and with the loving force that is the ultimate source of creation. This world Kabbalah terms the Tree of Life Reality.

I knew from my study of quantum physics that some scientists had already begun to postulate the existence of parallel universes as the only possible explanation for the results of certain laboratory experiments. Such leading theoretical physicists as Nobel Prize—winner Richard Feynman, David Deutsch, and Hugh Everett III had suggested that multiple possibilities co-exist simultaneously and, occasionally, intersect. These quantum physicists offered a view remarkably similar to that described in the Zohar. No wonder this approach—labeled "mystical" by those who didn't understand it—once had to be hidden from popular view!

As early as the 1950s, Everett had even coined the phrase "choice points" to indicate the points at which parallel universes were most likely to intersect with our own. At last I understood the meaning of the puzzling verses in Isaiah: "Seek God when He can be found. Call upon him when He is near." On a logical level, this made no sense. Wasn't God always available, always near? Yet the verse became stunningly clear if I read it as a reference to choice points, those key moments when our own limited material universe intersects with that parallel universe in which we are all united with the Creator.

The kabbalists not only knew about choice points, they were even able to tell us when they occurred. I learned that during certain times of the year, we had access to a choice point, such as the period of time known as the Days of Awe, from Rosh Hashanah, the Jewish New Year, through Yom Kippur, the Day of Atonement. These were times in the cosmic calendar when other worlds were particularly available to us—information that would obviously be quite useful to anyone interested in healing. We also experience choice points on a daily basis, for every encounter with another human being is a choice point, offering us the opportunity for profound spiritual growth.

The Zohar further explained that the Torah—the first five books of the Bible, in the so-called Old Testament—is actually replete with coded prophecies and a technology that we can use to remove suffering and find fulfillment. This coded wisdom enables us to tap into the power of the universe and gain access to profound wisdom, albeit in a highly concealed form. When I read *Cracking the Bible Code* by Jeffrey Satinover, M.D., a book detailing the Torah's prophecies, I found still more scientific and mathematical confirmation of the principles of Kabbalah.

MATRIX HEALING: A NEW KIND OF MEDICINE

Darkness cannot drive out darkness, only Light can do that.
Hatred cannot drive out hate, only love can do that.

—MARTIN LUTHER KING JR.

As I began to grasp the principles of Kabbalah, I felt an enormous sense of relief. At last, it seemed, my soul's hunger had been satisfied. Finally, I had discovered the ultimate integration of science and religion. Through my twin studies of Kabbalah and quantum physics, I, like Tipler, began to see that the spiritual principles of Kabbalah were not simply compatible with science but were themselves the best kind of science, that cutting-edge theoretical physics led right to the insights of the Zohar.

Through the prism of the Zohar I was able to understand that each of us has the power to choose life and health. If death and disease exist, it's only because we haven't yet understood that power—haven't yet mastered the software, so to speak, that would enable us to access it.

But I was a physician who had taken an oath to heal the sick. How could I integrate the amazing body of technological knowledge amassed by Western medicine with the profound insights of the physicists and the kabbalists? What new kinds of healing might be possible for mind and body, soul and spirit, if I could bring these worlds together?

Even as I wrestled with these questions, I had already begun sharing the kabbalistic perspective with my patients. How could I not? Here was the very hope they had been looking for, the very sense of empowerment that would enable them to heal themselves. Looking for a language that integrated the worlds of Kabbalah and science, I came up with the notion of the Matrix to express the kabbalistic notion of the Tree of Life—the parallel universe in which we are all already perfectly healthy, filled with the Light of the Creator. Accessing this Matrix involves a blend of physical and spiritual actions, based on the software outlined in the Zohar and other kabbalistic texts. Understanding the Matrix draws on both the spiritual wisdom of Kabbalah and the cutting-edge science of quantum physics, mind-body medicine, and the latest discoveries in anatomy, biochemistry, and neurology.

Modern medicine focuses on the darkness of disease. We analyze the darkness; we X-ray and scan it. We cut it out and irradiate it and throw one drug after another at it. Yet as Martin Luther King Jr. pointed out, darkness can never drive out darkness. Only light can do that. So I began to share with my patients what I knew about the Light.

When I tell my patients about the Matrix, I see their faces light up and their souls quicken. What a joy to be able to share with them this approach to life and health, and to watch them make dramatic—even miraculous—improvements in body, mind, soul, and spirit. Using the techniques of Matrix Healing, I've seen people recover from cancer, heart disease, and other severe illnesses.

Recently, for example, I treated a 44-year-old man who was HIV-positive. He took conventional medications but also undertook the meditations I suggested, read the Zohar—in itself a healing experience—and worked in various ways with the element of water, a powerful tool in Matrix Healing. Within a few months, we saw his viral load go down and his general health improve. Today he is living fully, enjoying his life, despite his ongoing HIV status.

Or consider the patient who was also a friend, a woman in her thirties with melanoma. Working with affirmations, meditation, and water, she achieved a complete spontaneous remission that I would have considered a miracle before I became a Matrix Healer. Now, of course, I've come to expect astonishing results from this extraordinary healing technology.

Matrix Healing is not only a matter of physical health. As my patients have applied the techniques I describe in this book, I've seen them transform their lives, choosing new possibilities in love, work, and family, as well as finding a new joy and vitality in their daily existence.

In this book, I share with you both the philosophy that underlies Matrix Healing and the practical steps you can take to access your own state of perfect health. In Chapter 1, I explain the scientific foundation for this view, while in Chapter 2, I lay out the basic premises of Kabbalah. The rest of the book offers insight into various aspects of health and healing. Chapter 3 explains the kabbalistic notion of *Sefirot*—energy centers that exist simultaneously within the body and the soul. In Chapter 4, we look at Matrix Anatomy, drawing upon both kabbalistic tradition and the latest discoveries in medicine for a new view of the human body. Chapter 5 shares the principles of Matrix Nutrition, an approach to food that integrates body and soul, while in Chapter 6 you'll learn about the healing properties of water. In Chapter 7, I help you see how every moment of your life can be an opportunity for greater health and happiness, a way of accessing what I call "doses of spontaneous remission." Chapter 8 explains the ultimate Matrix software, the techniques for meditation and prayer that can help you achieve mind over matter. And in Chapter 9, I share my sense of the grand ecology of our universe—the way in which we are all part of one another, our planet, and the divine.

THE JOY OF HEALING

> I will give you a new heart and put a new spirit in you. I will take from you the heart of stone and give you a heart of flesh.
>
> —EZEKIEL

What I share with my patients—and what I'd like to share with you—is both the secrets of Matrix Healing and the sense of excitement that this new worldview has brought me. When I think of the Matrix, I seem to experience quite literally the new heart and spirit promised by this verse from Ezekiel. And it takes so little to start the journey! Just one moment of acting differently from how we normally would, just one charitable action or empowered choice, and suddenly a whole new world opens up. As the Zohar says, "Open to me an opening no bigger than the eye of an needle, and I will open to you the heavenly gates."

So welcome to the Matrix! I hope that you, too, will encounter these ideas as an opening of the heavenly gates, enabling you to enter a hitherto unsuspected world of healing, health, and joy.

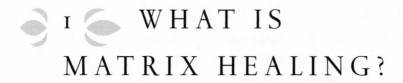

1   WHAT IS MATRIX HEALING?

I'LL never forget the first time I met Joan, a patient who had come to me after being diagnosed with an advanced form of breast cancer. Joan was a shy, quiet woman in her early fifties, dressed in a light gray suit and dark blue blouse. The only touch of color in her outfit was a small yellow enamel pin in the shape of a daffodil, pinned to her lapel. There was something about the image of the little flower, alone against the expanse of pale gray cloth, that I found both moving and painful.

Like many of my patients, Joan had been to a number of other doctors before she'd come to me. She'd already had a double mastectomy and subsequent treatments of chemotherapy. But, as sometimes happens, the cancer had come back. Joan had heard about my efforts to integrate a spiritual perspective with the latest in medical care, and she thought such an approach might help her defeat the disease that seemed so determined to remain with her.

As we spoke, I was struck by the way every aspect of Joan's life seemed to come down to two unpleasant choices. As a young woman, she'd had the chance to take an exciting job in another city. But she worried that such a choice might disrupt her relationship with her fiancé, who was just getting started in his own career, so she turned the job down. Later, after she'd gone back to college to become a social worker, she decided that she wanted to get further training in psychoanalysis and become a private therapist. By the time I met her, she had successfully completed her training and established her career—but now she was haunted by the worry that her demanding practice was depriving her three children of her time, energy, and attention.

So when Joan asked me to tell her how Matrix Healing might apply to her situation, I found myself telling her the story of the man and his dream. "That's the perspective that Matrix Healing can offer," I explained. "Most of us have an outlook on life that is far too limited. But Matrix Healing can help us wake up to all sorts of new possibilities."

Joan was intrigued by the concept of the Matrix—the parallel reality that each of us can access right here and now. A rational person with a strong faith in science, she was drawn to this vision of science and spirituality coming together, supported by the latest research in quantum physics, neurology, psychology, and medicine. She began to see that this research all pointed in the same direction: to the notion that we human beings have far more control over our bodies, our health, and our lives than most of us ever suspected.

NEW FRONTIERS IN SCIENCE AND HEALTH

> [A]lthough quantum physics supplanted classical physics a
> century ago, the implications of the quantum revolution
> have yet to penetrate biology and in particular, neuro-
> science.
>
> —JEFFREY SCHWARTZ, M.D., AND SHARON BEGLEY,
> *THE MIND AND THE BRAIN*

When I was in medical school, all my professors agreed absolutely: there was the human body, and then there was the reality "out there." Things from "out there"—germs, bacteria,
viruses—invaded our individual bodies, causing illness. More
things from "out there"—drugs, medicine, surgery—could penetrate us "in here," curing illness. Both getting sick and getting
well were seen as purely objective processes that could be measured, quantified, and, eventually, controlled.

Although doctors might disagree on this or that cure, they all
agreed on one thing: the patient's own consciousness was irrelevant. What mattered was the doctor's ability to manipulate drugs
and body parts, much as a mechanic manipulates the parts of a
car. It would be a foolish mechanic, indeed, who believed that his
or her feelings—let alone the car's feelings!—had anything to do
with getting the vehicle back on the road. We doctors were considered equally foolish to believe that either our own or the
patient's consciousness played any role in the healing process.
Yet, as we saw in the Introduction, this vision of the body as
machine was based on a long-outdated model of the physical
world, grounded in the seventeenth-century classical physics
proposed by Sir Isaac Newton and supplemented by the mechanistic views of René Descartes.

Ironically, there is some evidence that Newton studied Kabbalah and that, on a personal level, he had a spiritual, almost mystical, view of the universe. Certainly, he was a great scientist, the founder of modern physics, discoverer of the laws of motion, the force of gravity, and the basic principles of thermodynamics.

Yet almost despite himself, Newton's scientific approach introduced into Western thought a problematic, even destructive tendency. Particularly as taken up by Descartes, Newton's genius inadvertently led Europeans to the gradual adoption of a mechanistic worldview.

Before Newton and Descartes, the world seemed to be full of mysterious forces—some spiritual, some physical, and all poorly understood. The new science they stood for offered another view of the world—as a vast machine, operating according to the natural laws of gravity and magnetism. In this world, material forces were responsible for everything that happened. If we used the scientific method to conduct well-organized experiments, we could observe and measure those forces. If the experiments were conducted properly, they would always come out the same way, no matter which scientist was in charge—and no matter what the individual scientist felt, believed, or expected.

The separation of consciousness from the material world was central to this new idea of science. What an individual scientist believed wasn't supposed to matter: well-run experiments should always produce the same results. You might be Christian while I was Jewish; you might be an atheist while I was a believer; you might agree with Newton while I disagreed—no matter. Our consciousness was irrelevant. Only the physical world was important.

Medical science adapted this model for the human body. During the Middle Ages, humans were seen as a mysterious mixture of physical and spiritual, body and soul, animal and divine. But as the so-called scientific approach caught on, doctors started to view human beings in purely physical forms. An individual doctor might believe in God or in some spiritual principle—that was his or her own business. But such opinions had nothing to do with the pure science of medicine.

This approach led to an entirely new way of viewing the human body. Traditional medicine had seen the heart, for instance, as a place where spiritual and physical functions joined, and doctors as well as poets had spoken of the heart as the seat of love. But in the spirit of the new science, the pioneering British anatomist Thomas Harvey argued that the heart was simply a mechanical device, a pump whose primary function was to distribute blood throughout the body. To Harvey and his followers, the poets were silly dreamers, while the new doctors were practical men of science.

To be fair, a great deal of good came out of this mechanistic view. Scientists who saw the heart as a pump went on to invent new types of heart medicine, open-heart surgery, pacemakers, and all sorts of other technological wonders. I'll be the first to admit that modern medical technology has saved thousands, if not millions, of lives. Certainly, I myself rely on modern technology in countless ways as I treat my patients.

Nevertheless, an overreliance on technology and the mechanistic worldview that created it has led to a medical science that is simply incorrect. Harvey's important discoveries notwithstanding, we now have access to scientific data of a very different kind. We know that anger, worry, and anxiety are bad for the heart. And recent research has shown that whenever we experience love, caring, and compassion, the heart's electromagnetic coherence increases and its health improves. Apparently, the ancients were right: we do indeed love with our hearts. (For more specific information on these ideas, see Chapters 4 and 7.)

Another limitation in medical science comes from the tradition of basing all medical knowledge on studies of the corpse. Again, dissecting cadavers has led to enormous advances in medical science. But it has also limited our understanding in crucial ways. After all, the human body is *not* a corpse. The effects of life—electromagnetic impulses, the impact of muscle movement on our mood, and a thousand other vital signs—simply cannot be understood by studying dead bodies. I vividly recall my own discomfort when I met my first cadaver in medical school. I wasn't put off by the formaldehyde or the rigor mortis but rather by my growing realization that here was where modern medicine was looking for its answers—in bodies that literally lacked thoughts, emotions, and souls. The logical outcome of this approach was succinctly stated by the 1965 Nobel Prize–winning biologist Jacques Monod: "Anything can be reduced to simple, obvious, mechanical interactions."

QUANTUM MEDICINE

As the noted scholar Rabbi Elimelech reached the end of his life, he grew ill and was unable to eat. One day his son, Rabbi Elazar, begged him to take a little nourishment. "Oh," said Rabbi Elimelech, "I remember once I was in a little village, staying in the local inn. I had the most marvelous soup—it tasted delicious, like paradise! Never in my life have I had a soup like that."

Rabbi Elimelech died at his appointed time—but many years later, his son happened to be in the same village, staying at the same inn. Remembering what his father had told him, he asked the hostess for some of her special soup. "All I have is beans and flour," the woman told Rabbi Elazar, "which is not nearly good enough for a *tzaddik*—a saint—like yourself. But I will make you a bean soup if you like."

When Rabbi Elazar tasted the woman's bean soup, he thought he was in paradise. "My father was quite right, this is delicious!" he told the woman. "What did you put in the soup besides beans?"

The woman began to cry. "I have nothing, nothing but beans and water. As I began to cook the soup, I prayed to God: 'Master of the Universe, I have nothing but beans and water—but you have access to *Gan Eden,* to Paradise, where all the scents and flavors of the universe may be found. Take some of those scents and flavors, and put them in my soup, so this good man can have the meal that he deserves.'"

—TRADITIONAL CHASIDIC TALE, ADAPTED WITH PERMISSION
FROM *NOT JUST STORIES*, RABBI ABRAHAM J. TWERSKI, M.D.,
ART SCROLL/MESORAH PUBLICATIONS

In the mechanistic worldview of Descartes or Monod, a story like this Chasidic tale would be considered the essence of irrationality. If two different cooks are given the same beans and water, the same pots, and the same stove, then both soups should taste exactly the same, regardless of the attitude of the cook.

But in the early twentieth century, Albert Einstein and his colleagues had already begun to suspect that this mechanistic view was radically incomplete. These groundbreaking scientists proposed a challenging new vision of the universe, known as quantum physics, which began to blur the boundaries between observer and observed, mind and matter, intention and result. Suddenly, it seemed that our consciousness of the world might actually help shape reality.

Today's quantum physicists might view Elazar's story with a bit more sympathy. To the modern scientist, the consciousness of the observer can indeed affect reality, just as the consciousness of the innkeeper affected her soup.

Welcome to the Matrix! In the participatory universe revealed by quantum physics, our consciousness can actually *change* the material world—including our bodies and our state of health.

The notion that consciousness can affect reality was first put forward by nuclear physicist Werner Heisenberg, author of the famous Heisenberg uncertainty principle. The details of Heisenberg's argument are too complicated to go into here; suffice it to say that Heisenberg and many scientists who came after him believed that the very process of observing reality actually transforms that reality. Specifically, Heisenberg demonstrated that there is no way to observe subatomic particles without the very process of observation affecting the particles' behavior.

Heisenberg also argued—through a complicated set of mathematical equations that I won't reproduce here—that our observation actually enables us to create new realities. Thus, he and his colleagues believed, subatomic particles exist only when we observe them, that our observation of these particles literally brings them into existence, much as the innkeeper's vision of paradise literally brought into existence the heavenly flavor of her soup.

Lots of people have had trouble with this hypothesis, including the father of modern physics, Albert Einstein himself. But even Einstein agreed that Heisenberg's argument made sense. And today, most physicists do accept Heisenberg's arguments.

"I think we have long since passed the place in high energy physics where we're examining the structure of a passive universe," says physicist Robert G. Jahn, as quoted in Michael Talbot's fascinating book, *The Holographic Universe*. "I think we're into the domain where the interplay of consciousness in the environment is taking place on such a primary scale that we are indeed creating reality by any reasonable definition of the term."

Jahn is no mystic. He's a professor of aerospace sciences and dean emeritus of Princeton University's School of Engineering and Applied Science, as well as a former consultant for NASA and the Department of Defense. He and his associate, clinical psychologist Brenda Dunne, conducted a set of experiments at the Princeton Engineering Anomalies Research Lab (PEAR), which Jahn founded in 1979.

In one notable experiment, Jahn and Dunne had volunteers sit in front of a type of computer called a random event generator (REG), a machine that generates a random sequence of numbers. After hundreds of sessions with volunteers, Jahn and Dunne discovered that almost every person involved in their experiment was able to affect the sequence of the REG's output simply by concentrating on the outcome he or she desired. Apparently, the volunteers' thoughts were literally transforming the operation of the machine.

Jahn and Dunne also had volunteers sit in front of another device, which distributed 9,000 ¾-inch marbles into nineteen collecting bins, much like a giant pinball machine. The laws of probability would indicate that these marbles should fall into a huge bell curve. But the volunteers were able to affect the patterns into which the balls fell to a small but statistically significant degree. These experiments strengthened Jahn's conviction that our consciousness literally enables us to affect different aspects of our world.

According to Jahn and Dunne, we may be able to create the results that we desire—or, in some cases, the results that we expect. We have probably all experienced something like this on a psychological level. Most of us know people who expect to be given special treatment, and for no apparent reason, they seem to get it every time. Likewise, we may have noticed that when we're in a bad mood, everything that happens seems to confirm our sense that life is rotten, whereas in a happier mood, we experience one piece of good fortune after another.

Jahn and Dunne have evidence for this principle on a subatomic level. In the late 1980s, physicists discovered a particle whose behavior was so idiosyncratic that they actually called it the *anomalon*. This anomalous particle seemed to behave differently in different laboratories, as though the expectations of the physicists who studied it were literally affecting its behavior.

Likewise, in the 1930s, the physicist Wolfgang Pauli was trying to solve a particular problem concerning radioactivity. He suggested that the problem could be solved if we assumed the existence of a subatomic particle without mass, which he called the *neutrino*. Sure enough, in 1957, scientists found evidence for a massless particle, which they called the neutrino.

Then some other physicists pointed out that a neutrino *with* mass would help solve several other problems—and so in 1980, laboratories in the Soviet Union began finding evidence of neutrinos with mass. U.S. labs, meanwhile, found no such evidence. Finally, in the late 1980s, some labs outside the Soviet Union were able to duplicate the Soviet findings—but others were not. Once again, different observers seemed to be getting different results. Could it be that these highly trained scientists were simply doing the experiments "wrong"? Or was it possible that different expectations enable us to access different realities, just as Heisenberg had suggested?

Jahn and Dunne believe that these contradictory findings are evidence that Heisenberg was right: that our expectations literally help us create different versions of reality. It's not just a question of bias—that we focus on what we're looking for and simply ignore the rest. Our thoughts, feelings, and beliefs actually shape the material world, including our own bodies.

CHOOSING AMONG PARALLEL UNIVERSES

All matter originates and exists only by virtue of a force, which brings the particle of an atom to vibration and holds this most minute solar system of the atom together. . . . We must assume behind this force the existence of a conscious and intelligent mind. This mind is the Matrix of all matter.

–MAX PLANCK, QUANTUM PHYSICIST

As you can see from the Max Planck quote, theoretical physicists were being pushed—often against their will—to advocate theories that previous generations of scientists would have pooh-poohed as the fantastic speculations that belonged more properly in books of fairy tales than in scientific journals. One of these fantastic notions, now accepted by a number of respected scholars, is the notion of parallel universes—other worlds that exist alongside our own.

One of the best-known scientists to put forth this possibility was Hugh Everett III, who in 1957 published a famous paper called "Relative State Formulation of Quantum Mechanics." There he coined the term *choice points,* those moments when parallel universes have the chance to intersect. In other words, choice points are those times when we have the opportunity to download another world.

Another famous advocate of parallel universes is the British scientist David Deutsch. In one experiment, Deutsch shot out a stream of electrons, trying to force them through one of two slits he had set up. Although the electrons, of course, remained invisible, Deutsch was able to see trace patterns of the electrons' path. He expected the electrons to travel in relatively straight lines, but instead he discovered an interference pattern that radiated outward, like the ripples in a pond. A huge number of "excess electrons" seemed to be crowding their way through the slits, a phenomenon that Deutsch could explain only by postulating an infinite number of "virtual electrons"—subatomic particles from a parallel universe. These virtual electrons had apparently interfered with the path of the actual electron, suggesting that parallel universes really do affect our own.

Deutsch's work remains controversial, though many skeptics admit that his is the best explanation so far for the phenomenon he has observed. To me, Deutsch's work offers further support for the notion that we can access many different universes, including the world of perfect health and fulfillment promised by Kabbalah.

THE Z-EFFECT:
FREEZING REALITY THROUGH OUR EXPECTATIONS

> Oh, ye terrestrial beings, who are sunk deep in slumber—
> awake!
>
> —THE ZOHAR

There is one more aspect of quantum physics that I'd like to share with you: the Zeno effect, or Z-effect for short, proposed in 1977 by physicist George Sudarshan of the University of Texas at Austin. Atoms and subatomic particles are usually in a state of flux, shifting from one energy level to another and back again. But Sudarshan found that if scientists observe an atomic system frequently enough, the very process of observation seems to freeze the system, holding it indefinitely at the same level of energy.

Sudarshan named his discovery after Zeno of Elea, a Greek philosopher who loved to propose paradoxes. But I like the Z-effect's nickname—"the watched pot effect." Apparently, in the world of quantum physics, a watched pot *literally* never boils! The simple process of "watching the pot" is enough to keep the pot in the same state of energy.

One of the most striking confirmations of the Z-effect, as reported in *The Mind and the Brain,* by Jeffrey Schwartz, M.D., and Sharon Begley, came from a 1990 study conducted at the National Institute of Standards and Technology (NIST). Researchers at NIST observed beryllium ions, measuring the chances that these unstable entities would decay from a high-energy to a low-energy state. They found one level of probability when they measured the ions infrequently. But the more they measured and observed, the less likely the ions were to decay. Repeated observation seemed literally to freeze the ions into a high-energy state. Or to put it in another way, continually focusing on one property of the ions—their energy level—seemed to prevent the ions from being able to change.

When I explained this idea to my patient Joan, she was amazed.

"In other words," she said slowly, "focusing on my cancer has actually 'frozen' the disease into my body. The more attention I've given this disease—the more often I've thought about it, or been tested for it, or wondered whether it's gone away—the more I've actually been ensuring that it stays inside of me."

"Well, there's no scientific evidence to apply the Z-effect to disease—at least, not yet," I replied. "But I personally believe that the process you just described is exactly the way our bodies work. After all, why should our bodies operate by different laws than subatomic particles? Focusing on a problem just reinforces that problem. Our challenge is to focus not on disease, but on health and full recovery—which, by the way, is a principle that Kabbalah teaches, as well."

This conversation proved to be a real turning point for Joan. She took to heart my suggestion that she "wake up" from her dream of a limited world into a more accurate perception of the limitless possibilities that life had to offer her. She began to realize that according to both Kabbalah and science, there was a new world before her, with a reality that was quite different from the one in which she had been led to believe. I could see in her eyes that her soul had started to quicken as she realized that she literally had the power to access a new reality and create miracles.

Meanwhile, Joan was undergoing a number of treatments that I had prescribed. In addition to the standard chemotherapy that virtually every breast-cancer patient receives, I was helping Joan detoxify her body by altering her diet (for more on Matrix Nutrition, see Chapter 5) and exposing her to infrared rays. Hydrotherapy—alternating hot and cold baths—was also helpful (for more on the healing powers of water, see Chapter 6), as was Bikram yoga, a form of yoga practiced in the heat to encourage the body to sweat.

I explained to Joan that we needed to address her body as well as her spiritual state, since when the temple that houses the soul is more purified, spiritual practices are more effective. But she was also praying and meditating (for more on prayer, see Chapter 8), accessing the "parallel universe" in which she was already healed.

Joan could immediately see the difference even in her experience of chemotherapy. She experienced far fewer side effects than she had before, retained her appetite—unusual for chemo patients—and even managed to keep most of her hair.

Meanwhile, Joan had gone on to make some major life changes. She restructured her practice as a therapist, moving into joint office space with a colleague with whom she could share referrals.

"Now I have more time to spend with my children, but it feels as though my practice is still operating at almost the same level," she told me. "I always thought I'd hate sharing an office, but I actually like it. Sharing space makes it easier to consult with a colleague when I need help. It makes the work less lonely, and I think I'm now more effective with the patients I do treat." Believing that life held new possibilities had actually helped Joan access those possibilities, just as the faith of the innkeeper in the Chasidic tale had enabled her to access the flavors of a heavenly soup.

THE MEDICINE OF SELF-EMPOWERMENT

> A doctor once went to see a patient who had been sick for a long time. "Let me explain something to you," he told the discouraged man. "In this room, there are three of us—you, me, and the disease. If you and I join forces, then we'll outnumber the disease two to one, and we have a good chance of winning. But if you join forces with the disease, that's two to one against me—and against *that* combination, my friend, I'm sure to lose!"
>
> —ADAPTED FROM BAR-HEBRAEUS, THIRTEENTH CENTURY, SYRIA; A VERSION OF THIS STORY APPEARS IN *A TREASURY OF JEWISH FOLKLORE*, EDITED BY NATHAN AUSUBEL

The doctor in this thirteenth-century story understood something very important about health and healing—something that has been confirmed by a number of medical studies: when people feel out of control, they often get sick. And when they feel empowered to choose for themselves, they are more likely to get better.

Remember, quantum physicists have already determined that we live in a participatory universe. When you participate fully—when you become master of your own ship, so to speak—you're more likely to heal.

The question of being "in control" or "out of control" is key to understanding something that has become almost a medical cliché in recent years—the notion of stress. Because of the way this issue has been reported in the media, many people have come to see stress as a bad thing, a factor in the development of heart disease, ulcers, migraine, colitis, and a number of other medical conditions. And indeed, stress can be an important factor in our health. For example, a Mayo Clinic study of people with heart disease found that psychological stress was the strongest predictor of future cardiac events, including cardiac arrests and heart attacks.

In the world of Matrix Healing, though, stress is not necessarily bad. *Stress* is just another word for challenges—new and unexpected demands made on our bodies and spirits by various life circumstances. Losing a job or having a loved one die can be a source of stress. So can getting a fabulous new promotion at work, falling in love, or even acquiring a beloved pet. Both positive and negative life events may demand a great deal from us—but they don't necessarily make us sick. In fact, some people seem to thrive on stress, becoming healthier and happier with each new challenge. What makes the difference?

According to a number of medical studies, a key factor in our health is our sense of control or self-empowerment. Simply getting stressed—or sick—as the thirteenth-century Syrian doctor knew, isn't enough to kill us. What's deadly is the sense that we have no ability to meet the challenge, that all we can do is lie back and let any unfortunate event assume power over our lives.

The importance of empowerment is strikingly demonstrated by a famous study in which rats were injected with a tumor preparation, giving them all an equal predisposition to develop cancer. Researchers then divided the rats into three groups. One group was simply left alone, in what we might consider the "no-stress" model of life. A second group was subjected to periodic, uncontrollable, inescapable electric shocks. A third group also received electric shocks, but was taught how to escape them.

The results are instructive. As we might expect, the most tumor-prone group was the one receiving inescapable shocks. Only 27 percent of the rats living that "high-stress" life rejected the tumors with which they had been implanted. Meanwhile, twice as many of the "no-stress" rats—54 percent—were able to reject the tumor. But here's the real surprise: an even higher number—63 percent—of the rats who received electric shock and learned how to escape it ended up cancer-free. Apparently, it's even more healthy to handle a stressful situation than it is to avoid it.

In a similar experiment, two groups of rats were given electric shocks at identical times. Rats in the first group, however, were taught that they could avoid the shocks by turning a little wheel in their cages. The second group was given no such option. Scientists found a considerable drop in the immune functions of the second, powerless group, while the "empowered" rats in the first group stayed healthy. Both rats were "stressed"—that is, shocked. But the rats who felt able to take control of their situation had stronger immune systems.

If control over stress is so important even to rats, how much more necessary is it to human beings? In a famous study conducted among executives at Illinois Bell Telephone, researchers queried some 800 middle- and upper-level executives at the phone company, having them fill out detailed questionnaires about stress and illness in their lives. Many of the executives described themselves as having high-stress lives, and indeed, many reported that they frequently got sick. Yet many others reported themselves as generally healthy. What distinguished the two groups?

Researchers suspected the differences might be based on such variables as age, income, or job level, but in fact, these factors played little role in people's health. Rather, the people who got sick least often—despite their admittedly high-stress jobs—were those describing themselves as more in control, more committed to their work, and more challenged. In other words, having a boring high-stress job was more likely to make people sick than a job that, while stressful, also seemed challenging. Likewise, a high-stress job that someone didn't really want could easily lead to stress-related illness, while having a high-stress job to which a person felt committed was a recipe for health.

Thus, researchers found that executives who approached their jobs with enthusiasm coped with stress much better than executives who felt tired, burned-out, and ultimately passive—not unlike the patient in Bar-Hebraeus's story. Likewise, executives' sense of control over their work and their lives was also an important factor. Executives in the "high-stress/low-illness" group made such statements as, "The policy comes down from above that I'd better change the makeup of my office, but how that's going to work is up to me." Like the rats who had learned to avoid electric shocks, executives who felt they had at least some choice, some control over their environment, tended to be healthier as well as happier.

But the most important factor in determining health,

researchers found, was the degree to which executives felt that they expressed themselves through their work. The executives who were getting sick had lost touch with their own values and priorities—or at least, they didn't feel that their jobs allowed them to pursue their personal goals. The executives who flourished in spite or even because of the stress experienced their jobs as fulfilling their commitment to themselves. They believed in what they were doing, and so they enjoyed the challenges rather than feeling overwhelmed by them.

The results of the Bell Telephone study have been supported by a huge body of other research. An international study of nearly 3,000 people between the ages of 55 and 85 found that people who felt in control of their lives had nearly 60 percent lower risk of death from any causes, compared with those who felt relatively helpless. Other studies have shown that the biggest single predictor of whether patients will survive their first heart attack is not cholesterol, diabetes, or high blood pressure, but job satisfaction.

But my favorite "empowerment" study is the simplest one of all. Some patients in an intensive care unit were given one very basic choice: what kind of sheets would be placed on their beds. Although most doctors I know would consider this detail a supremely unimportant aspect of health care, people's health improved when they were allowed to choose for themselves.

THE HEALING POWER OF COMPASSION

Some day after we have mastered the winds, the waves and gravity, we will harness for God the energies of love; and then for a second time in the history of the world, humans will have discovered fire.

—TEILHARD DE CHARDIN

So far, we've focused on the role of empowerment and control as elements of health. But just as important—perhaps ultimately more important—is a sense of compassion, an experience of being connected to other human beings, of caring for others and receiving their care in return. A 1995 study published in the *Study for the Advancement of Medicine,* for example, revealed that when patients experience compassion, their levels of salivary IgA—the body's first line of defense against viruses and other pathogens—increases significantly. A similar study by A. Thomas McLelland at Harvard University also showed that an experience of compassion raised sIgA—even in people who claimed to have no subjective feeling of compassion. (We'll look more closely at McLelland's studies and the research they inspired in Chapter 7.)

Compassion was certainly the key factor for E. Langer and J. Rodin, who in a 1976 study explored the effects of giving plants to nursing home residents. Some residents were told that their plants would be taken care of for them, while others were invited to care for their own plants. Within just a few weeks, residents who cared for their own plants showed a noticeable improvement in physical and psychological well-being, and had also become more active than the patients whose plants were cared for by others. Most astonishing, however, was the long-term follow-up, which found that eighteen months later, patients caring for their own plants had a mortality rate only half that of the control group. Clearly, offering compassion—even to plants—gave a significant boost to patients' health.

Researchers such as Dean Ornish, M.D., have long argued for the importance of social connection as a factor in health. Ornish, author of *Love and Survival: The Scientific Basis for the Healing Power of Intimacy,* has written, "People who volunteer to help others also greatly increase their health and survival. Investigators have found that activities involving regular volunteer work were among the most powerful predictors of reduced mortality rates."

Likewise, psychologist Stephanie Brown of the University of Michigan Institute for Social Research conducted a 2002 study in which she found that when the elderly offer social support to friends, relatives, and neighbors, they can lower their risk of premature death by 60 percent. "These findings suggest that it isn't what we get from relationships that makes contact with others so beneficial," Brown commented. "It's what we give."

Brown's work is supported by numerous other studies, including one conducted by Liang Krause Bennet, published in 2001 in the journal *Psychology and Aging,* and a 1998 review of seven studies on the relationship between volunteer work and health, all of which demonstrate that volunteering is indeed good for your health.

Further evidence of the healing power of compassion comes from the Tenderloin Senior Outreach Program (TSOP), which set up a series of weekly support groups for elderly tenants of low-priced hotels in San Francisco's impoverished Tenderloin District. The support groups became action groups as tenants began working to solve the neighborhood problems they identified— crime, hunger, and the like. Residents from several local hotels founded the Safehouse Project, with nearby stores and businesses offering themselves as a haven where residents could go for help in an emergency. Formerly inactive elderly and impoverished residents of this low-income and dangerous neighborhood went on to organize successful campaigns to block illegal rent increases and to feed the hungry in their community. "For many," wrote Professor of Public Health Meredith Minkler in her account of the project,

involvement with TSOP led to increased self-esteem, [a] . . . sense
of control . . . and a sense of connection with others that previously
had been missing. One elderly tenant, a former resident of a state
mental hospital, captured this change succinctly. Norris had been
in the habit of making monthly visits to the state mental hospital
for reality orientation, but after two years' involvement with TSOP,
the visits stopped altogether. When asked about this he replied,
"I'm a co-leader of my hotel support group, a founder of the
anticrime project, and a member of the Mayor's Task Force on
Aging. I don't have time for reality."

From her observation of TSOP, Minkler concluded, "Being
meaningfully involved with others, deriving the support that
comes from giving and seeking assistance, and feeling increased
control as a consequence can have powerful health effects." Or,
in Matrix Healing terms, having opportunities to show compassion and feeling empowered to make changes in one's community are good for your health.

MATRIX HEALING AND KABBALAH

Once a woman went to the Rabbi of Belz to ask him to pray
for her health. Her legs were badly swollen, and no doctor
had been able to help her. But the rabbi's study was so
crowded that the poor woman could not enter, so she went
to ask the rabbi's wife for help in reaching the rabbi. "He
certainly won't be able to see you today," said the rabbi's
wife, "but I'll tell you what to do: add another candle to the
Sabbath lights and that will heal you." The woman was
indeed healed, which she later reported to the rabbi.
      "Whatever gave you that idea?" the rabbi asked.
      His wife smiled. "In Tehillim [Psalms 119:105] it says, 'Your

word [of Torah] is a lamp for my feet.' And we know that
Torah can heal. So I knew that adding holy light would help
heal her feet."

—TRADITIONAL CHASIDIC TALE, ADAPTED WITH PERMISSION
FROM *NOT JUST STORIES*, RABBI ABRAHAM J. TWERSKI, M.D.,
ARTSCROLL/MESORAH PUBLICATIONS

So far, we've looked at Matrix Healing from a purely scientific
point of view. But, although I am a scientist, I am also a believer
in the Torah and the Zohar. Like the rabbi's wife, I believe that
their words have enormous healing power—a power that even
the quantum physicists have barely begun to suspect.

I wanted this to be a practical book, and so I've included many
specific precepts about how to live a healthy life: how to eat,
breathe, and meditate; how to draw on the healing power of
water; how to attune your life to the rhythms of the cosmic calendar. The practices in this book will work for you, whether or
not you share my belief in Kabbalah. But I believe with absolute
certainty that, like the extra Sabbath light in the story, understanding Kabbalah can bring a healing power into your life
beyond anything you can imagine. In this chapter, we have seen
that there is a scientific foundation for the principles of Kabbalah.
In the next chapter, we'll begin to explore Kabbalah itself. But
first, as a taste of the kind of Matrix Healing work I do with my
patients, here's a meditation that can help you get in touch with
your sense of empowerment and creativity.

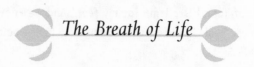

The Breath of Life

PREPARATION

1. Begin by setting aside 15 minutes for this exercise. As you become more used to meditating, work your way up to 30 minutes.

2. Sit in a comfortable position with your back straight and your feet flat on the floor. Don't fold your hands or cross your feet—you'll learn in Chapter 3 why it's important to allow the right and left parts of your body to remain separate.

MEDITATION

1. Breathe in slowly, on a count of eight. Don't force your breath; simply allow the breath to expand your diaphragm.

2. Now exhale, slowly, on a count of eight. As you release your breath, connect to the image of the Creator breathing life into the universe. Allow yourself to consider the possibility that you could have the same creative power within your own life.

3. Once again, breathe in slowly. Connect to the realization that the whole world was animated by the Creator's breath. Remember that every time you breathe, you're tapping into the cosmic creative process. As you release the breath, experience your creative power to bring new life into the world.

4. Continue to breathe in and out, knowing that you are tapping into the cosmic process of creation. Experience the way each breath brings the healing power of order and creativity into your life.

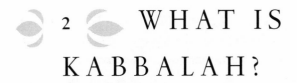

2 WHAT IS KABBALAH?

THE TORAH—

See, I have set before you life and death;
therefore, choose life.

WHEN Mitchell walked into my office, he had reached the end of his rope. A businessman in his late sixties, he'd been diagnosed with lung cancer about a year before. He had already been treated with chemotherapy, which had proved unsuccessful. He then moved on to another doctor, who had prescribed a new, experimental drug—also a failure. By now, the cancer had metastasized, and according to conventional medical wisdom, Mitchell had very little reason to hope.

"I've heard you specialize in unconventional treatments," he said to me. "I've never gone in for that sort of thing, but at this point, I'll try anything."

"Look," I said, "the only unconventional thing about me is that I believe you can be healed. The Light wants to enter your body—but *you* have to open the door. Is that something you're ready to do?"

I went on to explain that the kabbalistic image of Light is a metaphor for the deepest good in the cosmos—a way of indicating Divine Presence, Transcendence, Mystery, or what Kabbalah calls the Source of Sources. According to Kabbalah, I told him, that goodness wants to come into our lives, and with its help, we can heal any problem—emotional, physical, or spiritual.

"This I know," I told him, "as much as I know that penicillin kills bacteria. But whether or not you benefit from that goodness—well, that's up to you."

Mitchell looked startled. Whatever else he'd been expecting, clearly it wasn't this. "That's not what my other doctors have told me," he said skeptically.

I shared with Mitchell my favorite quotation from the Zohar, the 2,000-year-old book on which Kabbalah is based: "Open to me an opening no bigger than the eye of a needle, and I will open to you the heavenly gates. Thou art the door through which there is entrance to Me; if you openest not, I am closed."

"You're the door, Mitchell," I told him. "You can open to the Light or to the Infinite Presence, or whatever word you choose to refer to the Source of Sources, or God—or not, as you choose. Your health is entirely in your own hands."

Mitchell still looked skeptical, but now he also looked interested. "I don't know exactly what you mean by 'opening to the Light,'" he told me, "but at this point, I'm desperate. Whatever you've got, let's give it a try."

KABBALAH'S KEYS TO HEALTH AND HAPPINESS

The true value of a human being is determined primarily by the measure and the sense in which he has attained liberation from the self.

—ALBERT EINSTEIN

Over the past several years, I've seen how useful Kabbalah has been, in my life and in the lives of my patients. I've had firsthand experience of how this ancient wisdom has exponentially expanded both my own and my patients' capacity to lead healthy, successful, and joyous lives. In Kabbalah, I've come to believe, are the real secrets of health and healing, the true "medicine of meaning" that I've been seeking ever since I first became a doctor.

Certainly, a kabbalistic approach paid off for Mitchell. Of course, my treatment of him relied in part on standard medical practice. I'd just read about a new protocol for chemotherapy that had proved somewhat successful with his type of cancer, and we decided to start him on that. I also prescribed nutritional supplements that would boost his levels of albumen, decrease his production of insulin, and raise his secretory IgA levels. But most important, I wanted Mitchell to understand what I'd meant by "opening the door." I told him that for the first time in two thousand years, the wisdom of Kabbalah had become available to us all. Now we could learn the secrets that only sages, mystics, and prophets had known before, secrets that could help us access the Light. Kabbalah teaches that the Light *wants* to enter us—but we have to open up to it.

This approach has profound implications for treating diseases such as cancer. After all, why irradiate the darkness when you can just turn on the Light? If I could help Mitchell make room within himself for more Light, I believed he could be healed.

Kabbalah makes several specific suggestions for how we can open ourselves to the Source of Sources:

- **Develop a sharing consciousness.** According to Kabbalah, there are two basic ways to approach our lives: through ego, or with a sharing consciousness. While an ego-based approach may feel good in the short run, we can ultimately find health and happiness only when we share. God desires to give to us in ever-increasing amounts, but we make room for this bounty only when we give of ourselves.

- **Switch from a reactive to a proactive consciousness.** Kabbalah teaches that there are two forces operating within us—reactive and proactive, corresponding to two competing souls, the godly soul and the lower soul. Our reactive natures respond impulsively with a host of troubling emotions: fear, anger, greed, envy, hatred, apathy, frustration, and the like. These are expressions of the lower soul. Our proactive natures, coming from our godly soul, evoke quite different responses: compassion, serenity, charity, joy, trust, and a commitment to the greater good. Each moment, we have the opportunity to choose between these two souls, to give in to our reactive natures or to move forward with our proactive selves. Each time we resist the lower soul and tap into our godly soul—even if it's only to smile at a neighbor or hold the door for a stranger— we're giving ourselves tiny, potent doses of spontaneous remission.

- **"Give until you feel it."** Kabbalah tells us that "Charity can save you from death." In my experience as a physician, this is literally true, as medically sound a statement as "Lowering blood pressure reduces the risk of heart disease" or "Breakfast is the most important meal of the day." If you give away a significant amount—not the giving that is easy to do, but an amount of money, time, or effort that really constitutes giving of yourself—your health will improve.

- **Become absolutely certain that you are already healthy.** Once we comprehend that it is in our natures to be healthy, happy, and filled with Light, we begin to view our health with certainty. We don't just hope to be healed. We understand on the deepest level that we are *already* healed, that our illness and discomfort are simply distortions of the Tree of Life reality. If we decide to choose the Matrix and the Tree of Life, health and happiness lie within our grasp. At every moment of our lives, the choice is up to us.

In other words, every time we do something proactive, we overcome our reactive natures, even if only for an instant. At that moment, the Light—the creative force of the universe—enters into the deepest recesses of our cells and begins the healing process at the most fundamental level.

ENTERING THE MATRIX

A change in meaning is a change of being.

—DAVID BOEHM, QUANTUM PHYSICIST

In our first few appointments, I shared a kabbalistic approach with Mitchell, explaining to him the principles of Matrix Healing. I told him that somewhere buried deep within the self he recognized was another person—a proactive, sharing person who was free from the desire to receive for the self alone. That proactive person was already healed, and if Mitchell could access that deeper self, he could overcome his cancer.

Somewhat to my surprise, Mitchell grasped these concepts right away. Perhaps his years in business had taught him what a big difference the right attitude could make, how much power each of us has to change our world. Or maybe he was just ready to hear something new. Either way, he began to practice the meditations I suggested for him. Slowly but surely, he started to view himself as a being who confronted every obstacle with an ever-greater determination to choose proactively. He began to see himself as a spiritual vessel whose very nature was to receive larger and larger shares of Light. And he understood that the way to expand his vessel was by making proactive choices, creating more room to let in more Light.

Mitchell also took several specific actions. He started drinking eight to twelve glasses of water a day, meditating each time he drank on the theme of "being like water." In Kabbalah, water represents the ultimate "sharing consciousness," seeking only to give of itself, flowing wherever it is needed, sustaining all life on earth. Trying to "be like water" is one way to expand our own ability to share. (For more on the healing element of water, see Chapter 6.)

Mitchell also took seriously Kabbalah's prescription of charity. He began giving away a substantial portion of his income—not the relatively small tax-deductible gifts he'd made in the past, but a genuinely significant piece of his wealth. "Give until you feel it," I reminded him, and Mitchell took me seriously. Much to his surprise, he found that the more he gave, the more his business—and his income—grew. The more he gave, the more he had to give—and the more his health improved.

But Mitchell didn't only give of his possessions. He also gave of himself. Around the time he began coming to me, a friend of his became very sick. Previously, Mitchell might have responded with an occasional visit, card, or phone call, especially since he himself was so sick, but now he decided to spend a great deal of time with his friend. He listened to his friend's fears and regrets, he was there through his friend's tears, his dread of the unknown, his dark night of the soul. For the first time in his life, Mitchell found himself focusing not on his own concerns but on the needs of another. I believe that caring is what finally galvanized his recovery.

To Mitchell's astonishment, his experience of chemotherapy

under my care was significantly different from any of his previous treatments, with markedly fewer ill effects and substantially more progress. Two years later, the tumor in Mitchell's lung had shrunk significantly—a most unusual result for someone with metastatic cancer. Indeed, only a small percentage of people with Mitchell's diagnosis survive for even two years. Mitchell had not only survived, he was living as a healthy man, continuing to prosper in his business, expand his philanthropic efforts, and enjoy all aspects of his life. Mitchell had truly made an opening within himself—and he felt as though he'd walked through the heavenly gates.

KABBALAH AND MATRIX HEALING

> A rabbi fell asleep and dreamed that he had entered Paradise. There, to his surprise, he found the sages discussing a knotty problem in the Talmud. "Is this the reward of Paradise?" cried the rabbi. "Why, they did the very same thing on earth!"
>
> Then the rabbi heard a scolding voice: "You foolish man! You think the sages are in Paradise. It's just the opposite! Paradise is in the sages."
>
> —JEWISH FOLKTALE, ADAPTED FROM *A TREASURY OF JEWISH FOLKLORE*, EDITED BY NATHAN AUSUBEL

When I first began to study Kabbalah, I was particularly intrigued by the notion of the parallel universe that it promised—what I've come to call the Matrix. In the Matrix, we are *already* healed, just as the folktale explains: paradise is already within us. Learning how to access this paradise is the secret of Matrix Healing.

Imagine a multiplex movie theater. Side by side many different movies are playing. While you're watching the movie in Theater 1, you have the sense that it's the only show in town. The movie (if it's any good!) takes you over completely, dominating your thoughts and emotions, catching you up in the problems and possibilities that it presents.

But suppose you decide to walk out of the horror film in Theater 1 and catch the comedy in Theater 2. Now you're in a completely different world, with different rules and parameters, different possibilities, a world that evokes thoughts and feelings you could barely imagine while you were sitting quietly in Theater 1. And all it took was walking from one movie theater to another.

I believe that with the right spiritual tools—meditation, understanding, and the daily practice of compassion and proactive responses—we can learn to access different versions of reality as easily as we might enter and leave a movie theater. And we can choose to enter the movie entitled *Perfect Health* whenever our bodies require healing.

Of course, the material world has its own reality. Living in this world, we can feel overwhelmed by the presence of death and disease, by the existence of evil, by the forces that work against our bodies and our souls. But, as Mitchell discovered, an endlessly abundant supply of Light is available to us all—if only we know how to access it.

The image of the movie theater is my own. Yet there's a whole body of medical research that supports this notion of parallel states of health and disease. For example, people afflicted with multiple-personality disorder might experience two, three, or more personalities within the same physical body—each with its own individual state of health. Supposedly incurable disorders such as hypertension or diabetes that plague one personality disappear within minutes when another personality takes over.

Some researchers have even found that wounds that were open and bleeding in one personality close up and heal for another, only to reopen when the first personality returns.

Of course, multiple-personality disorder is a serious psychological problem. But let's look for a moment at the implications it has for those of us who are not afflicted with it. Studies have found that when people switch personalities, their brain-wave patterns actually shift. Their capacities shift as well, with one personality speaking several foreign languages, even as another can barely put together a coherent English sentence. Or perhaps one personality is a talented artist while another has no interest or ability in painting. How many of us supposedly healthy people are harboring within ourselves "other personalities" with hitherto untapped capacities, powers of which we know nothing simply because they don't fit into our limited ideas of who we are?

Moreover, according to Dr. Bennett Braun, of the International Society for the Study of Multiple Personality, in Chicago, medical conditions can literally alter as various personalities shift. Braun reported one man who was generally allergic to orange juice, breaking out into a painful rash after even a small sip. However, one of the man's personalities was free from the allergy, and when that personality was in control, the man could drink as much orange juice as he liked. Even more dramatically, the rash he had acquired while the other personalities were in control began to fade as soon as the nonallergic personality took over. In Matrix Healing terms, it was as though he had simply stepped from one movie theater into the next, from the "allergic" movie in Theater 1 to the "allergy-free" movie in Theater 2.

Sometimes, the experience of multiples reminds us that we can access sickness as well as health. Dr. Francine Howland, a Yale psychiatrist who specializes in the treatment of people with multiple-personality disorders, once treated a patient who had been stung by a wasp. The man showed up for an appointment with his eye swollen shut, complaining of severe pain from the sting. As it would be some time before the ophthalmologist was available, Howland helped the man switch to an alternate personality, one that she called an "anesthetic" personality because it felt no pain. Within an hour the man's pain was gone and the swelling was gone, as well. Suddenly, there was no need for a trip to the eye doctor.

After he returned home, the man's other personality reasserted itself—and with it, the sensitivity to pain reemerged. His eye swelled up again, as though it had resumed the "ordinary" course of illness that had been interrupted when the second personality took over. Although the man hadn't needed medical treatment while the "anesthetic" personality was in control, his other personality desperately required the attentions of an ophthalmologist.

It's a well-known fact that tolerance for drugs varies widely among most people, based on age, body weight, personality type, and a host of other factors. Likewise, because of their lower body weight, children need smaller doses of drugs than do adults. But what happens when multiple personalities are prescribed drugs or given anesthesia? Doctors and anesthetists have reported numerous problems, since the dose that works for one personality may be too strong or weak for another. Some medicated adult patients suddenly manifest the symptoms of an overdose when they switch to a child's personality.

Clearly, our beliefs about who we are have a profound effect on how we relate to our bodies, our health, and our medical treatment. These effects appear even more dramatic when we consider multiple personalities with more severe disorders. In a 1985 *New York Times* article, for example, psychologist Daniel Goleman reported the case of a woman with multiple-personality disorder whose diabetes was so severe she had to go to the hospital. But when she switched personalities, her symptoms disappeared. Other observers have noted that epilepsy and even tumors may come and go as personalities change.

After my experience with Mitchell and other patients, these accounts don't surprise me at all. They fit perfectly with my understanding that paradise is within us—our only obstacle is not knowing it's there. And once we become convinced that sickness is our lot in life, you can be sure that we *will* get sick. The power of our mind is so great that it can create diabetic symptoms as well as remove them; it can summon an allergy complete with swelling and rashes, or consign that same allergy to oblivion; it can even call forth tumors and then make them disappear.

People with multiple personalities suffer intensely from their condition, undergoing years of therapy to heal their mental state. Yet even after they are pronounced "cured," they tend to retain their ability to switch out of medical symptoms virtually at will. As Michael Talbot notes in *The Holographic Universe,* "This suggests that somewhere in our psyches we *all* have the ability to control these things."

The question, of course, is how to tap into this remarkable power. The answer lies in Kabbalah, whose potent technology enables each of us to access our own healing powers.

THE KABBALAH AND HOLISTIC MEDICINE

> Rabbi Tanhum once displeased a powerful Emperor, who had him thrown into a pen of wild beasts as punishment. The holy man had absolute certainty in the benevolence of God, and so the beasts did him no injury. Everyone who saw the rabbi emerge unharmed marveled at the miracle.
>
> But within the crowd was a man who had no faith in mir-

acles. "There's a perfectly simple explanation," he said scornfully. "The wild beasts simply weren't hungry—that's why they didn't eat the Jew!"

"All right," said the Emperor, "let's put your words to the test." He had the man thrown into the pen—and immediately, he was devoured.

—ADAPTED FROM THE *AGADA* IN THE TALMUD,
FROM THE VERSION FOUND IN *A TREASURY OF
JEWISH FOLKLORE*, EDITED BY NATHAN AUSUBEL

If Kabbalah is correct, if the data on multiple-personality disorders are correct, if quantum physics and its research on the power of our minds are correct, then why do we not all have perfect health? Indeed, why is the very opposite true? Why is the world wracked by new pandemics? Why are the U.S. rates of cancer skyrocketing? Why are Americans becoming less and less healthy, more prone to obesity, heart failure, stress-related illnesses, and other medical problems, even as we spend billions of dollars on health care and vastly increase our intake of medication?

I'm going to make a suggestion here that might have gotten me thrown out of medical school. Yet I believe with all my heart that this is a *scientific* statement that should be adopted by all responsible physicians: Western medicine itself, with its materialistic focus on the body and its insistence on ignoring the spirit, is literally making us sick—and then is making it virtually impossible for us to heal.

I love the Talmudic story of Rabbi Tanhum because I think it makes the principle so clear: if you believe that you live in a world where wild beasts can devour you, then of course they will. And if you live in a world that accepts the power of cancer to kill you and sees a difficult course of chemotherapy as your only option, then that's the reality you will experience.

But if you *know* that your true self is always protected—if you know that within the Matrix, on the spirit level, you are always safe and healthy—then, like Rabbi Tanhum, you can emerge unharmed. Everything depends on the power of our *certainty,* the ideas that we know to be true.

For this reason, the healing suggestions in this book are organized somewhat differently from those in a standard medical text. In the conventional medical approach—known as *allopathic medicine*—specific medicines are prescribed for particular problems. Cancer, heart disease, diabetes, and depression are all regarded as separate syndromes, each with its own specific medical protocol. As we saw in Chapter 1, the attitudes of patient and physician are irrelevant in this view.

A kabbalistic approach, by contrast, is holistic, considering the human body as a single system and viewing the mind, soul, and spirit as integral parts of that system. As a result, conditions that in Western medicine would require separate treatments might with a kabbalistic approach all be treated the same way. Mitchell, for example, suffered from lung cancer, and I suggested that he meditate, practice charity, and "be like water." But I've often given similar advice to patients with asthma, a heart condition, or gastrointestinal problems.

Rather than focusing on body parts and diseases, Kabbalah emphasizes the need to understand ourselves and our place in the universe. Each of us has different strengths and weaknesses, and we all have our own spiritual lessons to learn. But I believe it's far more profitable to focus on those lessons than to restrict our inquiry to individual disorders. So without disregarding the contributions of Western medicine, I want to emphasize the spiritual approach. As Mitchell learned, once we master the right outlook, the effect of any other treatment can be multiplied a thousandfold.

THE BASIC PRECEPTS OF KABBALAH

The great sage Rabbi Yohanan ben Zakkai once asked his five disciples, "What is the most desirable thing to strive for in life?"

Rabbi Eliezer said: "A good eye."

Rabbi Joshua said: "A good friend."

Rabbi Yose said: "A good neighbor."

Rabbi Simeon said: "Wisdom to foretell the future."

Rabbi Eleazar said: "A good heart."

"The words of Eleazar please me most," said Rabbi Yohanan, "because his thought includes all the rest."

—ADAPTED FROM THE *AGADA* IN THE TALMUD,
FROM THE VERSION FOUND IN *A TREASURY OF
JEWISH FOLKLORE*, EDITED BY NATHAN AUSUBEL

Once we know that the Matrix exists, how do we access it? In my opinion, there are two ways.

One option is simply to follow the advice of Rabbi Eleazar and open your heart. If you practice true charity, with no benefit to the ego; if you seek to replace reactive responses like anger and greed with proactive choices like generosity and compassion; if you "become like the Creator" by giving unconditionally, then you are on the road to perfect health. In fact, every moment of charity, compassion, and appreciation is a tiny dose of spontaneous remission. Each time you replace a reactive response

("Don't bother me!") with a proactive choice ("I'll help you!"), you're improving your health.

But if you're like most of us, you'll probably encounter obstacles in your efforts to open up your heart. You may find yourself frustrated by your shortcomings or discouraged that your efforts to develop "a good heart" don't always work out as well as you'd like. You may even decide that it's too painful to think about your life in these terms, that the very promise of Kabbalah mocks you with your own limitations.

If that's the case, then don't despair. In Kabbalah, the goal is not to *be* perfect but to *become* perfect. We're all here to overcome our own limitations, and so every moment we're given an opportunity to move closer to the Light. To help us on our journey, Kabbalah offers us many unique and powerful keys. Here are just a few:

- Balance your *Sefirot*—the ten vessels of energy located throughout your body.

- Learn to see your body in spiritual as well as physical terms.

- Tap into the healing power of food through conscious eating and soulful nutrition.

- Take part in the sharing consciousness of water.

- Become "like the Creator," replacing reactive responses with proactive choices every moment of the day, seeing every moment as a spiritual opportunity.

- Employ the healing software of prayer, meditation, and the Hebrew alphabet—according to Kabbalah, the building blocks of the universe.

- Take your place as a loving, responsible member of the human race within the new ecology of the spirit, recognizing how we are all interconnected.

You can read more about each of these principles in the next seven chapters. First, though, I want to share with you the basic premises of Kabbalah, so you can see how your individual efforts fit into the grand story of the universe itself.

THE WORLD ACCORDING TO KABBALAH

If the doors of perception were cleansed, everything would appear to man as it is, infinite.

—WILLIAM BLAKE

Kabbalah's view of the creation of the universe is remarkably like that of modern physicists. As with many contemporary scientists, kabbalists believe the world started with a Big Bang.

But what came before the Bang? Physics has no answer to that question—but Kabbalah does. In the beginning, says Kabbalah, was an infinite force of pure, loving energy, which many kabbalists call "the Endless Light." This energy sought only to give, to share; but when all the world was giving, who was there to receive?

So the Light created a Vessel. Now, instead of one force in the universe, there were two: the Desire to Share, and the Desire to Receive.

The Vessel represented the Desire to Receive. Yet, created by the Light, it also resembled the Light. According to Yehuda Berg, author of *The Power of Kabbalah,* we might think of the Vessel as a cup carved out of ice. If we imagine pouring water into this cup, we can see a separation—the hard ice cup and the soft flowing water that fills it. But fundamentally, both cup and water are the same entity—H_2O. Likewise, Berg explains, the Light and the Vessel were made of the same substance, albeit in different forms.

So for a while, all was perfect harmony. The Light poured out its infinite bounty, and the Vessel enjoyed an infinite capacity to receive it all. This was true paradise, represented in the Old Testament as the Garden of Eden.

Eventually, though, the Vessel grew frustrated with its role. After all, it had been made by the Light, and so it resembled the Light. The Light was the cause, the source, the generous giver—and the Vessel wanted to share those properties. Like a well-loved child who suddenly wants to give Mommy and Daddy a present, the Vessel wished not only to receive but also to give. And, like a child who wants to decide things for him- or herself, the Vessel desired the power of choice. Suddenly, the Vessel wanted to become godlike—wanted, indeed, to become God. It wanted to create its own fulfillment.

So, frustrated with its role as eternal receiver, the Vessel pushed back against the Light, and for just one moment, refused to receive. And that moment, according to Kabbalah, was the Big Bang, in which the material universe as we know it came into being. Remarkably, the kabbalists seemed to anticipate the findings of modern physics and astronomy—at a time when most scientists were mired in the thinking of Newton and Copernicus!

THE BREAD OF SHAME

> Once Rabbi Aharon of Premishlan was spending *Shabat* with the great Chassidic master Rabbi Elimelech. When they met, Rabbi Elimelech reproached Rabbi Aharon, saying, "The Prophet Elijah has complained to me that you have rejected

him. He descends all the way from Heaven to visit you, offering to enlighten you about the Torah, and yet he tells me that you send him away! How can you be so vain as to reject his lessons?"

Rabbi Aharon shook his head vigorously. "No," he said, "I refuse to receive enlightenment as a gift, even from the Prophet Elijah. We are told that the mitzvah—the blessing— lies not in *knowing* Torah, but in *studying* Torah. Any Torah knowledge that I acquire will be by my own efforts. That is the only way it will have any value."

—ADAPTED WITH PERMISSION FROM *NOT JUST STORIES*,
RABBI ABRAHAM J. TWERSKI, M.D.,
ARTSCROLL/MESORAH PUBLICATIONS

The story of Rabbi Aharon at first seems counterintuitive. If the great Prophet Elijah himself descended from Heaven to illuminate Rabbi Aharon's understanding, how could Rabbi Aharon refuse? Why would Rabbi Aharon prefer to gain Torah by his own efforts, particularly when he might have smaller and less satisfying results?

The answer lies in a concept that the kabbalists called *Bread of Shame*. They say that when we eat bread that has been given us, rather than bread that we have earned by our own efforts, it is tainted with shame, with a feeling of being inferior to the one who feeds us. This Bread of Shame is precisely what the Vessel rejected when it pushed back against the Light during the Big Bang.

So, like Rabbi Aharon, the Vessel declared its independence. In effect, the Vessel said, "I prefer free will and my own efforts to the boundless generosity of the Creator. True, this may cause suffering in the short run. But in the long run, it gives me the chance to become like God."

This chance to participate in the Creator's work, to become the creators of our own lives, to fill ourselves with the godlike desire to give—this is the promise of Kabbalah. Rejecting the passive role of the eternal receiver, we opted for our own long, slow, and arduous process of evolution. Over countless centuries, we moved up the evolutionary scale from inchoate matter to plants, to animals, until finally we grew into human beings who might indeed become like God.

There is a wonderful quote from the Talmud that expresses this idea. First, the Talmud quotes the Bible verse that instructs us to "cleave to God." The Talmud goes on to ask, "How can one cleave to God? God is compared to a burning fire." And the Talmud answers: "Just as God is called merciful, so too you shall be merciful. Just as God shows loving kindness, so should you show loving kindness. Just as God buries the dead, so too you should bury the dead. Just as God visits the sick, so too you should visit the sick."

Thus, we can embrace God by becoming like God. Just as fire blends with fire, so can our loving, proactive natures blend with our Creator's nature. Eventually, Kabbalah predicts, we will all become one—with each other and with the Creator. The Vessel, created so long ago to receive, will blend with the Creator, finally capable of infinite sharing.

But because we are all part of the same universe, we're going to have to do it together. In Kabbalah, there's no such thing as an individual who "returns to God" while the rest of humanity languishes in misery and error. On one level we each have our individual destinies, our individual souls and bodies. But on a more profound level, we all partake of the same soul, the same body, the same Vessel, and the same Light. If disorder or violence exists anywhere in the world, then it will somehow find a way to lodge itself in every person's immune system. Our separateness is an illusion—but it is an illusion that we must overcome together.

OVERCOMING OUR REACTIVE NATURES

> Life is a spell so exquisite that everything conspires to break it.
>
> —EMILY DICKINSON

From a kabbalistic perspective, life is a constant battle between two forces. We've called those forces our reactive and proactive natures. We might also call them entropy (the tendency of things to fall apart) and complexity (the tendency of things to become more orderly and complex). Or, as the kabbalists do, we might use the code word *Satan* (pronounced Sah-TAHN) to indicate the reactive forces within us that are always conspiring to "break the spell" and sabotage our chances for perfect happiness.

According to Kabbalah, each obstacle in our lives—each illness, hardship, or loss—is there to tempt us to give in, to allow our reactive natures to take their course. On the other hand, each time we resist the negative force of Satan, making proactive choices and maintaining our certainty in the Light, we become more like the Light and our health improves.

As you can see, the kabbalists have no interest in a satanic devil carrying a pitchfork and sporting a pointy tail. Rather, kabbalists see *Satan* as a code word for our reactive natures. By not understanding the negative forces of Satan's continuous challenge to our proactive choices, we fall prey more easily to temptation.

I like to think of the Satan portrayed in one of my favorite Jewish jokes. In this story, Satan stalks angrily into God's hall of judgment and complains that he's bored. "But you have so much to do!" God protests. "Haven't I assigned you the very time-consuming job of leading humans into evil?"

"Hah!" snorts Satan, with a look of disgust. "That's no challenge. Before I have the chance to even say one little word, humans have already gone ahead and jumped into evil all by themselves, without any help from me!"

"RECEIVING FOR THE SAKE OF SHARING"

> See I have set before you life and death; therefore, choose life.
>
> —THE TORAH

Of course, it's giving in to Satan that makes us sick and unhappy. The road to health and fulfillment lies elsewhere—but only when we resist our satanic impulses.

The primary way that Satan manifests within us is through what the kabbalists call "the Desire to Receive for the Self Alone." This is the selfish desire we may have felt as children, when we were given a box of candy and wanted to eat every piece ourselves.

Now, there's nothing wrong with the act of receiving. In fact, our goal is to expand our Vessel so that we can receive ever-greater quantities of Light. But in order to expand our Vessel, we must first restrict it. Instead of giving in to our childlike impulse to keep everything for ourself, we might recall our pleasure in sharing good things with the people we love. Hoarding the candy feeds our reactive natures—our greed, fear, envy, and insecurity, our lack of trust in the universe to provide us with endless treats.

Sharing the candy supports our proactivity, reminding us that we live in a universe full of beloved people and infinite bounty.

So perhaps after an initial struggle, we restrict our Desire to Receive for the Self Alone and focus on the Desire to Share. We offer the candy to those around us, and take pleasure in their pleasure.

Suddenly, we've created a new consciousness—the Desire to Receive for the Sake of Sharing. This is the highest level of consciousness we can attain—and the one guaranteed to make us healthiest.

Here's a meditation that I share with my patients to help them activate this new consciousness, or to switch from reactive to proactive. It is based on a statement from the gospel of the Essenes, a religious community to which Jesus belonged: *In the moment between the Breathing In and the Breathing Out is hidden all the mysteries.*

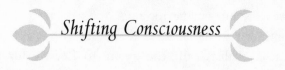

Shifting Consciousness

PREPARATION

1. You can do this exercise in 30 seconds, over the course of half an hour, or any time in between. It can help you through a stressful situation or simply remind you of what's most important in life.

2. If possible, sit in a comfortable position with your back straight and your feet flat on the floor. However you are positioned, however, don't fold your hands or cross your feet—you'll learn in Chapter 3 why it's important to allow the right and left parts of your body to remain separate.

MEDITATION

1. Breathe in slowly, on a count of eight. Don't force your breath; simply allow the breath to expand your diaphragm.

2. Now, for a moment, hold your breath. Recall that in the stillness between breaths, we have the opportunity to go from one consciousness to another.

3. As you exhale, releasing the breath from your body, visualize the Light flooding in where the breath used to be.

4. Say "Yahee," or "Let there be Light."

5. Even one deep breath can make a big difference, but feel free to repeat as often as you like.

THE KABBALISTIC HEALER

> What a piece of work is man!
>
> How noble in reason, how infinite in faculties . . .
>
> In action how like an angel
>
> In apprehension how like a god.
>
> The beauty of the world.
>
> —WILLIAM SHAKESPEARE, *HAMLET*

If I were invited tomorrow to address the American Medical Association (AMA), I would stand up before my fellow physicians and state confidently that the Light of healing and happiness is there in abundant supply—all we have to do is access it. I would cite the stories of Joan, and Mitchell, and many, many other patients as evidence of our universal ability to tap into the Matrix. I would even, perhaps, cite the quote from *Hamlet,* explaining that this view of humanity is not just optimistic poetry but, in my view, scientific fact.

"But if that's what you believe," I imagine one of my colleagues shouting out from the audience, "what do people need *us* for? If humans are godlike and the Light is endlessly available, why have healers in the first place?"

To answer this question, I would have to remind my colleague of the power of certainty. "Remember," I would say, "if people *know* that they can't achieve health, that life is dangerous, that the universe is stingy, then that is the reality they will inhabit. And since that is so often the case, our role as healers is to maintain the certainty of a better world. Our job is simply to *know* that the Light is infinitely available—and to help our patients know it, too."

Indeed, according to Kabbalah, God wants to give to us even more than we want to receive. This spiritual truth is expressed in the physical world as well, for as the Zohar says, the cow wants to nurse more than the calf wants to suck. Likewise, we often want more for our patients—and for our loved ones—than they are capable of wanting for themselves. In the same way, perhaps, the Creator looks at all of us, wanting only that we should accept the infinite Light and love that are available—and that we, in our smallness and ignorance, so often refuse to take.

Perhaps we push the Light away because we are afraid of our own greatness. Maybe on some level, we understand that giving and receiving so abundantly would indeed enable us to become gods. But our limited view of ourselves makes that kind of responsibility a frightening prospect. So we refuse the Light, even though accepting it would make us infinitely happier in the long run.

On a practical level, I can teach my patients some specific techniques for accessing the Light, techniques that I go on to share in this book. But on a more profound level, I think the kabbalistic healer is simply the person who reminds the rest of us who we really are: "In action how like an angel/In apprehension how like a god. The beauty of the world."

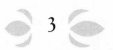 3   THE TREE OF LIFE: ARCHITECTURE OF THE SOUL

ADAPTED FROM THE MIDRASH, AND FROM *A TREASURY OF JEWISH FOLKLORE*, EDITED BY NATHAN AUSUBEL—

There was once a snake whose head and tail began to argue about their proper function in the snake's body.

"You're always out in front," the tail complained. "But I'm tired of letting you lead while I drag on behind! Let me lead, for once, and you follow."

The head agreed, and the tail began to lead. Soon they came to a muddy pit filled with thorns. As the tail had no eyes, it slithered right into the pit, and naturally, the head came, too. Both head and tail were slashed by the thorns, and the entire snake was grievously wounded.

Now, asks the Midrash, from which this tale is taken, who was to blame? True, the tail had insisted on going first. But what about the head— why did it allow itself to be led by a blind and brainless tail?

ANGELITA was a bright, ambitious woman in her late twenties. When she came to me as a patient, she was suffering from intense migraines that had started to strike with increasing frequency. As is common with migraine, the headaches had begun when Angelita was a teenager, and for several years, she had been using prescription medication to combat them. Now, however, her medication had stopped working. Although Angelita's previous doctor had offered to increase her dosage or perhaps find another prescription, Angelita herself was wary.

"My mother had migraines, too," she explained to me, "and that was her life for years—switching from one medication to another. Each new prescription worked for a while—and then, eventually, it stopped working and she had to switch again. I can see the pattern is already starting with me, and I don't want to go through all that. Is there anything else I can do?"

I explained to Angelita that migraines indicate a kind of imbalance in the circulatory system. Tension, certain foods, irregular sleep patterns, and a host of other triggers can cause the arteries to contract, depriving the vessels in the scalp of blood. Then, in reaction, the arteries fill up with blood too quickly in a rapid expansion that makes the vessels ache and throb.

As Angelita and I talked further, it became clear to me that her life seemed to mirror this lack of balance. She worked very hard all week as an accountant in a large corporation, a demanding job that called for her to come to work early each day and kept her at the office late each night. As a consequence, during the week she got very little sleep. Likewise, her high-pressure position made her too nervous to eat much, though she treated herself to a pastry or a brownie every evening as a bedtime snack.

Then, every Saturday, she collapsed, often with a migraine, sleeping long hours and doing very little. Each Sunday, she ran several miles, trying to burn off the sweet foods she'd been eating all week. Her intense schedule left her little time to socialize, though she was very involved with her family, who demanded that she come to her parents' house for Sunday dinner each week. This was basically the only social contact she had.

I made some basic suggestions to Angelita about diet, exercise, and lifestyle. Cutting back on her intake of sugar, regularizing her sleep patterns, and getting daily aerobic exercise—even if only a brisk 10-minute walk—would help address the physical side of her headaches. But I also suggested gently that other aspects in her life might be out of balance, as well. Perhaps, I told her, the headaches were her body and spirit's way of telling her that her energy wasn't flowing evenly throughout all the dimensions of her life. Perhaps, like the snake in the story, she was allowing certain aspects of her life to take the lead while neglecting other, more important dimensions.

"Maybe you're right," Angelita said doubtfully. "But then, what do I do about it?"

I thought Angelita would benefit from hearing about the kabbalistic view of how physical and spiritual energy flow throughout the body. So I began to explain to her the concept of the *Sefirot*. In Hebrew, *sefira* means "vessel," with the plural—vessels—being *sefirot*. According to Kabbalah, the *Sefirot* are ten vessels of divine energy that make up the Tree of Life. And when we learn how to balance our *Sefirot,* we are on the road to health.

THE *SEFIROT:* TEN ASPECTS OF BODY AND SOUL

> Now come and see the power of the righteous: they can
> unite all the sefirot, harmonizing the upper and the lower
> worlds.
>
> —CITED IN DANIEL CHANAN MATT,
> *THE ESSENTIAL KABBALAH:*
> *THE HEART OF JEWISH MYSTICISM*

As we saw in Chapter 2, there are two basic forces in the universe: the Light and the Vessel. The Light is the divine energy and love that emanate from the Creator—essentially, the Desire to Share. The Vessel is the entire material world and everything in it—all brought into existence in order to receive the Creator's Light—or in other words, the Desire to Receive.

In our earthly life, *Light* and *Vessel* are relative terms. When I'm giving, I'm the Light. When I'm receiving, I'm the Vessel. But whether it's coming through other humans or directly from the Source, Light is constantly available, in infinitely abundant amounts.

However, if we tried to receive the Light in our material form, it would literally "burn us out," overwhelming us with its power. Just as you can't plug a household lamp into an electric company's power station, so are we unable to receive the Light directly. There has to be a kind of filtering system, something that makes the Light available to us in a form that we can handle.

So according to Kabbalah, every Vessel is divided into ten *Sefirot.* Just as a prism divides white light into its many component colors, so do the *Sefirot* divide the Light into ten different aspects. Interestingly, string theory—one of the latest frontiers of quantum physics—has also recently suggested that the world is composed of ten dimensions, a scientific view that seems to echo the insights of the kabbalists.

These ten *Sefirot* are known collectively as the Tree of Life, after the tree in the biblical story of the Garden of Eden. According to Kabbalah, each of us has within us a Tree of Life that can indeed bring us eternal life, health, and happiness as soon as we learn to access the Light that filters through it. In Matrix Healing terms, we can enter the "movie" entitled *Tree of Life Consciousness* anytime we choose. We simply have to become aware of the ten *Sefirot* within us and balance the energy flowing within these spiritual and physical vessels. In kabbalistic tradition, the roots of the Tree of Life are in the *Ein Sof*—the "other realm"—that divine dimension where only Light exists. The Tree of Life grows from that dimension into this one, its heavenly roots drawing the Light of divine love into our bodies, minds, and spirits.

Thus, the goal of each "righteous" person is to keep energy continually flowing among our *Sefirot,* the ten smaller vessels that make up our larger vessel. Of course, to the kabbalists, *righteous* doesn't just mean "upright and moral." The word also indicates a healthy, happy, and fulfilled person, someone overflowing with love and joy, a proactive person who is constantly looking for new ways to share. Balanced *Sefirot* indicate that our energy is flowing freely, nourishing every aspect of our bodies, souls, minds, and spirits. Unbalanced *Sefirot* mean that we are suffering—physically, emotionally, spiritually, or several ways at once.

Although Angelita's Filipino family were all devout Catholics, she herself had become interested in Eastern religions. So when I told her about the *Sefirot,* she immediately thought of the chakras, the Hindu system of seven energy centers that rise in a straight line from the base of the spine to the crown of the head.

In many ways, the *Sefirot* do resemble the chakras. Each is a system of energy centers that we can identify physically throughout the body, but that also reveal the architecture of our minds, emotions, and souls. Each is a multidimensional approach to human life, in which body, mind, and spirit are intertwined.

Though similar, however, the two systems are not identical. Chakras are located in a single straight line from the base of the spine to the crown of the head. *Sefirot,* by contrast, are located in three columns—right, left, and central: in the crown of the head (central), over the two ears and in the two shoulders (right and left), over the heart (central), in the two hips (right and left), over the groin (central), and at the feet (central). (There is also an additional *Sefira,* not part of the original system but used by some kabbalists and healers, located in the throat, also in the central column.)

Recall how when we were first created, we were entirely made to receive the Creator's Light. Then, because we were made from the Creator, we became like the Creator, partaking of the Creator's Desire to Share. This dual nature is reflected in our *Sefirot:* the energy centers in our left column contain the Desire to Receive, while those in our right column embody the Desire to Share. Integrating the sharing and receiving energies of the right and left columns creates the powerful energy of the central column: the sharing, love, and continuity that becomes receiving *in order to* share. This is what the kabbalists call "Tree of Life consciousness" and what I call "living in the Matrix."

Thus, as we saw in Chapter 2, the truly healthy person fully experiences both the Desire to Receive and the Desire to Share, synthesizing them into a new balance. A child, for example, might be thrilled to receive a special birthday treat—but then takes pleasure in sharing that gift with brothers, sisters, and friends. Or a student might eagerly desire to receive knowledge—so that one day he or she can become a teacher and share that knowledge anew.

THE *SEFIROT* AND OUR HEALTH

> The opposite of a correct statement is a false statement,
> but the opposite of a profound truth may also be a pro-
> found truth.
>
> —NIELS BOHR

Angelita was interested in the *Sefirot* and the Tree of Life, but she didn't see what it had to do with her own health problems. So I told her the story of the snake from the Midrash. By the time the poor creature was in the thorny pit, I pointed out, it had clearly developed all sorts of health problems. Like most conventional Western doctors, I might begin treatment by addressing the most obvious symptoms: removing the thorns and prescribing antibiotics for the wounds. In the same way, I was happy to discuss with Angelita the physical approaches she might take to alleviate her migraines, which for a time might even include medication.

But clearly, if the snake continued to allow his tail to lead and his head to glide behind, his health problems would never stop. Sooner or later, he would glide blindly into another pit, or perhaps into an even greater danger. To really heal the snake, I would have to ask him why his head was so weak and his tail so strong. I would need to help him balance the energy of these two different aspects of himself, so that all aspects of his body, mind, and spirit could function as a harmonious whole. In the same way, for Angelita's headaches to really disappear, she might have to look beyond nutrition and exercise to deeper issues in her life.

Angelita understood the concept. She even agreed that perhaps her job and her family were taking up too much of her physical and emotional energy, and that she might benefit from a more balanced life. But as soon as we started talking about how she might achieve that balance, she came up with a thousand good reasons why nothing could change. She wasn't strong enough to stand up to her family; she would lose her job if she didn't work the long hours; she just "wasn't the type" to meet new people. The more we talked, the more helpless she felt. Soon, even giving up her bedtime snack and taking a daily 10-minute walk seemed beyond her resources.

"All right," I said finally. "Let's come at the problem another way. Forget everything else and concentrate on the *Sefirot* themselves. I have a feeling that once you really get in touch with the energy of these ten dimensions, the healing process will basically happen by itself."

Angelita agreed to spend 15 minutes each day thinking about her *Sefirot* and doing the meditations I taught her. Her goal, we agreed, was to become intimate with each one of her *Sefira* and to try to achieve balance among all ten. She also promised to try for just thirty days the changes in diet and exercise that I had suggested, and to keep a daily journal recording briefly what she ate, how long she slept, what kind of exercise she did, and how she felt that day.

As Angelita and I made her next appointment, I found myself wondering what the next month would bring for her. I knew that once people get in touch with the Tree of Life within them, they suddenly find themselves capable of making remarkable advances in health and healing—almost without effort. This to me is the power of Kabbalah: once you tap into the energy of the *Sefirot,* you discover that your body, mind, and spirit are all working together in a new way, generating a new level of health.

KETER: **THE CROWN**

> A person is neither a thing nor a process, but an opening or
> a clearing through which the absolute can manifest.
>
> —MARTIN HEIDEGGER

The first *Sefira* is called *Keter,* which means "crown." It is located at the top of the head—literally, at the crown of the skull—and it is the place through which divine Light filters into our material dimension. *Keter,* then, is a paradox—at once Light and Vessel.

Because *Keter* is the connection to the infinite, its nature is very difficult for us to grasp. In each of us, *Keter* represents the transition from nothingness to something, the moment when spiritual Light and energy penetrated into a new dimension to create the universe. If we picture the *Sefirot* as the Tree of Life, with its roots in heaven and its branches flowering throughout our bodies, we can see *Keter* as the place where the tree breaks through the earth, transmitting the energy of the roots into a healthy, growing plant.

Although some healers I know do a great deal of work with *Keter,* most kabbalists advise focusing on the other *Sefirot. Keter* is such a profound mystery that it may be enough simply to know it's there.

WISDOM AND UNDERSTANDING:
CHOCHMA AND *BINA*

> [Great poets can] by the pure and free exercise of their will
> reach a state in which they are at once cause and effect,
> subject and object, hypnotist and sleepwalker.
>
> —CHARLES BAUDELAIRE, *ON WINE AND HASHISH*

Chochma—the *Sefira* that surrounds the right brain—literally means "wisdom." It represents inspiration, the divine spark penetrating into our awareness. *Bina*—surrounding the left brain—means "understanding," though I prefer to think of it as "interpretation" or "translation." *Chochma* enables us to access new ideas, new ways of seeing the universe, new visions of ourselves and others. *Bina* helps us translate this insight into form, structure, words, mathematical formulas—whatever gives our initial inspiration enough shape and solidity to be communicated to others.

Over the past few decades, popular culture has included many references to the "right brain" and the "left brain." In popular terms, the right hemisphere of the brain is responsible for intuitive understanding, holistic appreciation of a problem, integrating many small details into a unified picture. The left hemisphere is supposed to be our analytical, logical, detail-oriented side, earthbound and practical. The right brain supposedly takes care of the whole, while the left brain focuses on the parts. The right brain is our connection to mysteries and inspiration, while the left brain lays out a problem clearly, with logical explanations.

As a doctor and a scientist, I'm uncomfortable with this literal view of the brain and its hemispheres. We know from people who have suffered strokes and other types of brain damage that the brain is an incredibly plastic and adaptable organ. Thus, when one region of the brain becomes unable to perform its functions, another region often takes over. I think it's a mistake to ascribe functions too literally to physical portions of our brain, given the evidence that so many of these mental tasks can be reassigned.

However, as a Matrix Healer, I know that the images of right and left brain are actually our attempt to indicate a deeper reality —the *Sefirot* of *Chochma* and *Bina*. In this view, *Chochma* is the initial inspiration, the "aha!" moment in which Mozart suddenly hears an entire symphony or when Newton finally grasps the law of gravity. *Bina* is the ability to translate this inspiration into concrete form—to actually write the notes of the symphony or lay out the mathematical formulas that explain the insight.

Let's look a bit more closely at *Chochma*, the *Sefira* that enables "divine inspiration." Artists and scientists have talked about such moments of vision, in which everything seems suddenly to become clear. Even people who reject traditional religion have described this experience of inspiration as allowing something larger than themselves to "work through them," of being given a gift or shown something by a higher power. In my opinion, they are describing the experience of *Chochma* as the divine Light channels its inspiration through this *Sefira*.

In some cases, the inspiration comes in the form of dreams. For example, Russian chemist Dmitri Mendeleyev reported in 1869 that his ability to lay out the Periodic Table of the Elements came from "a dream where all the elements fell into place as required." U.S. inventor Elias Howe dreamed of being chased by cannibals with spears, each spear bobbing up and down with a tiny hole in its blade. When Howe woke up, he realized that he had discovered the solution to his automatic sewing machine— he had to put the eye at the bottom of the needle, instead of at the top, as he had been doing. Danish physicist Niels Bohr described a dream of sitting on the sun, surrounded by planets whipping around him on tiny cords. This image led him to develop the model of the atom as a nucleus surrounded by orbiting electrons and other subatomic particles.

It's interesting to recall that the Greek view of inspiration was that of muses who whispered into the artist's ear. The artist's job was to translate these "musings" into poetry, architecture, or music, giving their divine inspiration an earthly form.

Of course, people who reject traditional religion might argue that inspiration and vision do not literally come from God or from a muse. The great psychologist Sigmund Freud long ago revealed that both dreams and artistic symbols can be viewed as products of our own minds—clues, images, and signs that we create and then reveal to ourselves. As in the quote from Charles Baudelaire, the great poet can be seen as both the hypnotist who gives the commands and the sleepwalker who carries them out. Both Freud and Baudelaire suggest that one part of our minds gives us a flash of insight or inspiration, which another part of our minds must then interpret, explain, or translate into concrete form.

As a Matrix Healer, I welcome this interpretation because it suggests what Kabbalah has long maintained: that we ourselves are in the process of becoming gods—creators who make beautiful worlds. When we tap into the *Sefirot,* we can reveal to ourselves and one another the divine wisdom that God is giving to us. In that view, artists and scientists are simply modeling for us on a grand scale the kind of divinely inspired discoveries that all of us are capable of making every day, every moment of our lives. In that view, *Chochma* is the *Sefira* that receives divine inspiration and helps us see things in a totally new way, to create new insight for ourselves and for each other.

Thus, even for those of us not currently engaged in ambitious artistic or scientific endeavors, *Chochma* is still a crucial part of our soul's architecture. It reminds us that we can always reenvision our lives, discover new ways of understanding ourselves and our world, and wake up into a new reality, simply through the power of *Chochma*. In Matrix Healing terms, *Chochma* is our ability to see an entirely new movie, to envision a more satisfying and healthy life for ourselves, to perceive possibilities and opportunities that we formerly could not imagine. *Chochma* represents our ability to start anew—to download a new reality.

BINA—UNDERSTANDING INSPIRATION

A young man once came proudly to a great rabbi and boasted about his saintly qualities. "I used to be an ordinary young man," he explained, "but then I was seized by the desire to become holy. Now I only wear white robes, the way the old sages used to. I never drink anything but water, and I mortify myself each day—putting nails in my shoes and lying naked in the snow. I even ask the *shammes* of my local synagogue to beat me every day, to express my penance for my sins."

The rabbi pointed to the white horse standing in the yard. "Look there, my son," he said. "That animal, too, wears spotless white, drinks only water, has nails in his shoes, rolls in the snow, and gets beaten every day. Now, I ask you—is it a saint, or is it a horse?!"

—JEWISH FOLKTALE, ADAPTED FROM
A TREASURY OF JEWISH FOLKLORE,
EDITED BY NATHAN AUSUBEL

Once we have envisioned some new possibility, how do we make it real? That's where *Bina* comes in. If *Chochma* represents the blinding moment of inspiration, *Bina* represents the many long and painstaking hours of translating that inspiration into a concrete form.

You may have experienced this process in your own life. You're facing a difficult problem at work or at home, and suddenly you have a flash of insight. You *know* how to solve the problem. The answer appears to you all at once, as a unified whole.

But you can't stop there. Now you have to find a way to put words to your idea, to mold your idea into something concrete and apply it in the real world. Somehow you must find a way of translating your flash of inspiration into solid, practical terms. That process of translation relies on the energy that comes from *Bina*.

Another aspect of *Bina* is interpretation. Without a correct interpretation, we are liable to misunderstand the inspiration we have received, to use it in the wrong way. Suppose you're driving your car down the highway and you hear a funny noise. No one else in the car can hear it, but you can, and you're sure that it indicates a problem. That little noise is like *Chochma,* the divine signal that provides you with mysterious new information.

So far, so good—but what does that little noise really mean? Perhaps your engine isn't working properly. Or might you have a problem with the transmission? Maybe one of your tires is low on air. Or could it just be a loose object banging around in the trunk? This is where *Bina* comes into play—the ability to interpret the mysterious signals of *Chochma,* translating them into useful, concrete information.

Religious stories and folktales from every tradition stress the importance of *Bina.* The divine prophecy is received from the oracle, only to be interpreted in the wrong way. A fairy tale describes a recipe for success, but only the hero can follow it. The tale of the saint and the horse is one of my favorite "*Bina* stories" because it shows how easily we can misinterpret divine commandments. The poor young man in the story once had a moment of inspiration that moved him to become more holy. But instead of finding a useful way of interpreting that insight, translating his divine inspiration into charitable deeds or genuine self-reflection, he chose a literal-minded and ultimately foolish interpretation of what might have been a flash of wisdom. In kabbalistic terms, he was lacking in *Bina*—his *Sefirot* were out of balance.

If I were diagnosing the young man in the story, I'd say that he was relying too heavily on *Chochma* at the expense of *Bina*. My patient Angelita seemed to have the opposite problem. Her practical understanding had helped her excel at work, manage her finances, and arrange the material side of her life. But she was missing a sense of inspiration, an openness to new ways of thinking about herself and her life. Her practical understanding was working within a very limited sphere, lacking the insight that might have enabled her to open up her life.

Both the young man and my patient might have benefited from a new intimacy with their *Sefirot,* and from creating a better sense of balance among them. Here is one of the meditations that I suggested to Angelita, to help her do just that:

 Balancing Chochma *and* Bina

PREPARATION

1. Set aside at least 15 minutes for this exercise—30 minutes is even better. Find a relatively quiet place where you won't be interrupted.

2. Sit in a comfortable position with your back straight and your feet flat on the floor. Don't lie down—you might fall asleep! Let your

hands rest loosely in your lap. Don't fold your hands or cross your feet—allow the right and left parts of your body to remain separate.

3. Close your eyes and take ten deep, slow breaths. Ideally, you should be breathing in on a slow count of eight and breathing out on the same count. If you find it difficult to breathe that slowly, work your way up to it, starting with a count of two, then four, then six, and finally eight. Don't force your breath. Allow it to float in slowly, gradually filling your diaphragm. Then allow it to float out in the same way, until every bit of it is gone. Your goal is first to completely fill your lungs and diaphragm with the breath, then to completely empty them—but this should feel effortless on your part.

4. Remember, every breath connects you with the creative power of the Creator, who first breathed life into the universe.

MEDITATION

1. Keep your eyes closed. Begin by visualizing *Chochma,* the vessel of energy around your right brain. Take some time to see it clearly, in your own way. You might picture a cup overflowing with water; a vessel full of light; a cloud of energy; a muse whispering in your ear; or any other image that works for you. As with your breathing, don't force or push anything. Allow an image to come to you and simply stay with it for a while.

2. When you have a clear image of *Chochma,* ask yourself to imagine this *Sefira* when it is in perfect balance. What color do you envision? What size? What intensity of light? Stay with the image until you have visualized a perfectly balanced *Chochma.*

3. Next, ask yourself what your *Chochma* looks like when it is too full—when its energy is dammed up and not allowed to flow freely into *Bina.* Again, visualize this image with as much detail as possible—color, shape, intensity, and any other details that come to you.

4. Now ask yourself what your *Chochma* looks like when it is "low"— when not enough energy is flowing freely into this vessel. Take your time. Notice every detail you can.

5. Finally, visualize once again your *Chochma* in perfect balance. Check in with yourself. Do you notice any differences in how your body feels with a balanced *Chochma*? What about your emotions? Your spirit? Rest for a moment with a perfectly balanced *Chochma* before going on to the next step.

6. Repeat the entire process with *Bina*. First, imagine what this *Sefira* looks like and feels like—maybe even what it sounds like. Does it have a color? A shape? Is it moving or still? Fixed or changing?

7. Once the image of *Bina* is clear, ask yourself to envision this *Sefira* in balance. Then, imagine excessive *Bina* that has been dammed up and not allowed to flow freely. Go on to visualize insufficient *Bina*. Finally, return to an image of *Bina* in perfect balance and rest with that image for a moment.

8. Now bring images of both *Sefirot* into your mind. Ask yourself to see your current state of *Chochma* and *Bina*. Pay attention to what you see in your mind's eye, without judgment or criticism. Are these two *Sefirot* in balance? Are both full of energy that flows freely? Or is there a block somewhere, an imbalance, excess, or insufficiency?

9. If you notice an imbalance of any kind, allow your mind to correct the problem. In your mind's eye, see the imbalance being rectified and harmony being restored. Visualize both *Chochma* and *Bina* strong and glowing—vessels of energy that flow freely throughout your body, emotions, and soul.

10. Take a moment to savor this image of perfect balance. As you continue to breathe deeply, allow your body to hold on to the sensations and emotions that accompany this balanced state. Remind yourself that whenever you feel "out of balance," you can

simply visualize this image once again—and instantly, your balance can be restored. Now, open your eyes.

DA'AT: TELLING THE WORLD WHAT YOU KNOW

The great Chasidic master Rabbi Elimelech once spoke to a group of listeners about the supreme importance of truth. According to the rabbi, a person who spoke only true words and not a single falsehood for only 24 hours was promised admittance into paradise—even if he or she were guilty of many other sins.

Shmuel the innkeeper heard the rabbi's words and decided to avail himself of what seemed like a relatively easy opportunity to assure himself eternal bliss. He told his wife to take care of the inn's business for an entire day while he shut himself into a back room, intending to remain alone for 24 hours. He even kept himself awake, fearful of talking in his sleep and perhaps uttering a lie.

Then, when only a few minutes of his 24 hours remained, Shmuel heard a loud knock at the door. The knocking was so insistent that he finally went to answer it, though he resolved to avoid speaking a falsehood at all costs. When he opened the door, he saw a peasant, who said, "I've come for my shovel, and now I want it back."

Shmuel was pleased at how easy it was to avoid a lie. "I've never seen you before," he said triumphantly. "And I certainly don't have your shovel."

"Yes, you do," the peasant insisted. "I left it here earlier today as a pledge for a drink I couldn't afford. Your wife told me to come back tonight with the money—and here I am!"

Sadly, Shmuel took the money and returned the shovel

to the peasant. Then he went to see Rabbi Elimelech and told him what had happened.

The rabbi smiled. "Now you see," he said, "that telling the truth is far more complicated than simply avoiding a lie. I never intended that you should isolate yourself from the world. If you really want to attain paradise, you have to speak the truth *with* people, not apart from them."

—ADAPTED WITH PERMISSION FROM *NOT JUST STORIES*,
RABBI ABRAHAM J. TWERSKI, M.D.,
ARTSCROLL/MESORAH PUBLICATIONS

Although the original set of *Sefirot* included only ten, some kabbalists refer to a new *Sefira, Da'at,* located just over the throat. If *Chochma* is where we give ourselves inspiration, and *Bina* is where we receive, interpret, and translate that inspiration into concrete thoughts and ideas, *Da'at*—literally "knowing"—is where we express that inner truth to the outer world.

Da'at is there to remind us that our inner truth is meant to be shared with others. As Shmuel learned, truth is not simply a matter of avoiding falsehood. Rather, truth is the responsibility to share our knowledge with the rest of the world.

Artists and scientists know how important *Da'at* is, and so they sculpt statues, compose symphonies, and publish research papers. The inspiration of *Chochma* and the understanding of *Bina* find their expression in the knowing—and speaking—of *Da'at.*

In *Da'at,* we also see the importance of the right, left, and central columns—the balance of sharing and receiving. Right-column *Chochma* shares with us the flash of insight that we need to see the world in a new way. Left-column *Bina* receives this inspiration and nurtures it with understanding. Finally, central-column *Da'at* produces a new synthesis: Receiving in Order to Share, speaking our new truth in order to share it with the world.

After all, what good is divine inspiration if we keep it to ourselves? How useful is a brilliant interpretation if no one else knows about it? *Da'at* reminds us that the ultimate purpose of *Chochma* and *Bina* is to share the fruits of our inspiration. Whether we're writing a poem, suggesting an improvement at our jobs, giving advice to a friend, or simply sharing our insights with those who are closest to us, *Da'at* energy is flowing. Likewise, when we refuse to share our truths with others, shutting ourselves away like Shmuel to avoid revealing our inner thoughts and feelings, our *Da'at* energy is blocked—and our spiritual, emotional, and perhaps even physical health will suffer.

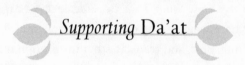

Supporting Da'at

PREPARATION

Use the same preparation described in the previous exercise.

MEDITATION

1. Keeping your eyes closed, allow yourself to focus on the sensations you feel in your throat. Is it scratchy and dry? Sore and swollen? Comfortable and relaxed? Without judgment or opinion, simply observe how your throat feels, in as much specific detail as possible.

2. Now allow yourself to visualize *Da'at*, the energy center located in your throat. What color is it? What size is it? Is the energy glowing and vital, or weak and depleted? Is the *Sefira* calm and balanced, or bursting with energy that has no outlet?

3. Imagine yourself restoring your *Da'at* to perfect balance. Visualize the right-column energy of *Chochma* and the left-column energy of *Bina* flowing into *Da'at*—two gorgeous streams of energy

nurturing this third *Sefira*. See your *Da'at* as a powerful but relaxed source of energy that fills your throat with healing light.

4. Now ask yourself what new truths you would like to express, using your new source of *Da'at* energy. Have you been avoiding a painful conversation with a loved one, or perhaps simply not expressing the depth of your love? Do you have an insight into your life that you've been ignoring because speaking from that place of truth might get you into trouble? Perhaps you simply have a creative new idea for making things go better at work or for beautifying your home. Visualize yourself pouring your own unique *Da'at* energy into the world—and see what happens.

CHESED AND *GEVURAH*:
REACHING OUT AND SETTING LIMITS

Jacob was a poor man who had always envied the wealth of others. Finally, he decided that he simply couldn't take it anymore. He went to the local rabbi to ask for the blessing of great wealth.

The rabbi looked thoughtfully at Jacob for a long time. Finally he said, "I will give you this blessing if you want it, Jacob, but first you must promise me something. Here are two gold coins. Use them to buy the finest food and wine. Then go home, and eat a wonderful banquet—by yourself. You must not share even a single morsel of food or a single drop of wine with your wife and children. Do I have your solemn promise?"

Jacob was puzzled, but he gave his promise. That night, he sat down to a magnificent table full of roast duck, wine, and other good things. He had expected to enjoy the food— his first taste of the wealth he desired—but then he noticed his wife and children watching him, silently, hungrily, with hollow eyes and sunken cheeks. Suddenly, every moment of the feast was torture. As he ate his way through the duck and drank his way through the wine, all Jacob could think of was how miserable his family looked, how hungry, how sick. If only he could share this feast with them—but the rabbi had forbidden it.

When Jacob returned to the rabbi, he was furious. "Why did you ask me to do such a terrible thing?!" he exploded. "That was the worst agony I've ever endured."

"Well," said the rabbi, "your family are not the only poor people in this town. Do you still want the blessing to achieve great wealth? Knowing that even as you and your family enjoy abundance, so many others are going hungry?"

"No," said Jacob. "Keep your blessing. If that's what wealth is, I don't want it."

From that day forth, Jacob's fortunes improved, and soon he became a wealthy man despite himself. But he never ate another meal at home. Instead, he gave generous donations to the town soup kitchen, and there he ate every day, along with the poor people who relied on his charity. He was no longer able to enjoy any blessing without knowing that he was indeed able to share it.

—FREELY ADAPTED WITH PERMISSION FROM
NOT JUST STORIES, RABBI ABRAHAM J. TWERSKI, M.D.,
ARTSCROLL/MESORAH PUBLICATIONS

The story of Jacob may seem extreme to many of us, but it illustrates an important kabbalistic principle: our profound need to give, share, and activate love. This need, too, is part of the architecture of our souls, as embodied in *Chesed*—loving kindness—

the *Sefira* located in the area of our right shoulder. Without the ability to give lovingly, our lives become barren and painful, no matter how much wealth, success, or popularity we enjoy.

The *Sefira* of *Chesed* embodies our deep desire to give, to contribute, to make a difference. Indeed, I believe that, ultimately, the greatest satisfaction we'll ever know comes from giving of ourselves—not simply donating money or even time, but truly sharing ourselves and our love with other human beings. This may take place on a personal level, between family, lovers, or friends. It may occur on a political level, as people like Martin Luther King Jr. or Gandhi shared themselves with the thousands of people inspired by their vision. Or it might be expressed through art or science, as writers, painters, and scholars pour themselves into their contributions—as I myself am trying to do, for example, by writing this book. No matter how we choose to do it, sharing ourselves with others is the most profound human experience we'll ever have.

And, as Jacob discovered, the contrary is also true: people who are unable to share themselves with others suffer the worst tortures of all. No matter how wealthy such people become, no matter how often they triumph over their enemies, no matter how much power they accumulate, it's never enough. They are tormented by the constant, nagging sense that they're missing something—and indeed they are. People who have been so abused or deprived that they are unable to care for others are cut off from their own *Chesed.* To be healed, they must reconnect to the power of this *Sefira,* to the loving, giving energy within themselves.

But simply giving because it makes us feel good is not necessarily helpful. Our giving must take place in a disciplined way, restricted to what is appropriate for the person who receives. Think of an alcoholic or a drug addict, desperate for a quick fix. If we impulsively give that person what he desires, it may make *us* feel better, but in the long run our gift will surely do more harm than good. Or imagine an enthusiastic fourth-grade teacher who offers college-level insight to her nine-year-old students. She may be inspired by a genuine desire to share her knowledge, but unless she restricts her giving to an appropriate level, her students are more likely to feel overwhelmed than enlightened.

These examples illustrate another important kabbalistic principle: the notion of restriction. As we've seen, the energy from a power plant must be restricted to flow through a system of wires and generators before it can usefully reach our homes. In the same way, the sharing energy of the right-column *Sefirot* must be restricted and governed by the receiving energy of the vessels in the left column. Thus, the right-column inspiration of *Chochma* must be channeled through the left-column interpretation of *Bina*. Likewise, the merciful *Chesed* energy in our right shoulder must be channeled through the severe judgment of *Gevurah*—the *Sefira* located in our left shoulder.

Chesed speaks to our wish to give, while *Gevurah* speaks to our good judgment and discipline. *Chesed* expresses our impulse to be instantly generous, while *Gevurah* reminds us to slow down and give at a pace we can sustain, in an amount that is appropriate to the person who receives. *Chesed* offers us the pleasure of abandoning ourselves to a cause or to another person whom we love. *Gevurah* reminds us to set boundaries, use judgment, and match our gift to the situation, not simply to our own impulsive wishes.

The tale of Jacob is a wonderful illustration of the importance of *Gevurah*. Clearly, the rabbi had the power to bestow upon Jacob the blessing of great wealth, but he restricted his giving, knowing that Jacob would benefit more if he received the blessing more slowly. Even the rabbi's first gift, the two gold coins, came with a limit: Jacob was permitted to use the money only to buy food for himself. What if the rabbi had simply given Jacob the money without restrictions? Jacob would have had the momentary pleasure of sharing a sumptuous dinner with his family, but he never would have learned the deeper lesson about his own need to express his *Chesed*. By giving too freely, the rabbi would have deprived Jacob of something he needed even more than the gold coins or the blessing.

It seemed to me that my patient Angelita suffered from an imbalance of *Chesed* and *Gevurah*, an imbalance that was making her migraines worse. On the one hand, she gave unstintingly to her job and her parents, putting in long hours at work and sacrificing every Sunday afternoon to attend the family dinner. On the other hand, she was receiving very little pleasure from either work or her family, and she had few other friends or loved ones with whom to share herself. Her sweet bedtime snacks were the only time she ever truly received something for herself—a dead-end kind of receiving that was also a powerful migraine trigger.

I hoped that by becoming more intimate with *Chesed* and *Gevurah*, allowing these energies to flow more freely, Angelita would both heal her migraines and improve her life. If you would also like a closer relationship with *Chesed* and *Gevurah*, use the *Chochma–Bina* exercise from the previous section, substituting *Chesed* and *Gevurah*. Only when both energies are flowing freely can we live healthy, loving, and self-loving lives.

TIFERET: THE BEAUTY OF A LOVING HEART

Beauty is truth, and truth beauty. That is all
Ye know on earth, and all ye need to know.

—JOHN KEATS

Tiferet literally means "beauty" or "splendor." It is the integration of *Chesed* and *Gevurah,* the place where giving and judgment join to express themselves in loving relationships.

Recall for a moment how the two streams of *Chochma* and *Bina* pour out through our throats into an expression of our inner truth, the *Sefira* of *Da'at.* In the same way, the mercy of *Chesed* and the judgment of *Gevurah* pour out through our hearts into a splendid expression of true love—*Tiferet.* Thus, *Tiferet* is both relationship energy and healing energy, the outward expression of *Chesed* and *Gevurah.*

Tiferet also means "truth," echoing John Keats's idea that beauty and truth are really aspects of the same quality. Whenever we see anything for what it truly is—seeing it fully, in all its unique splendor—we cannot fail to appreciate its beauty. This is as true for a stone, a tree, or a horse as it is for a human being: to see the entity's truth is also to see its beauty. This "true seeing" is the basis for authentic, loving relationships, in which giving and receiving are in balance, where love and caring are guided by judgment and discipline. In *Tiferet,* a perfect dynamic exists, and through this *Sifera,* life is experienced in the way it was intended—in true love.

As a central-column *Sefira, Tiferet* integrates sharing and receiving in a new way: receiving in order to share. This, too, is the basis for healthy relationships, in which both partners experience themselves as receiving even as they take pleasure in giving. Think of the child who insists on making Mommy or Daddy a birthday present. Now, consider the pleasure that the parents receive watching their child express such generosity. This is *Tiferet* energy, in which giving and receiving flow freely, creating loving, sharing relationships.

In the kabbalistic tradition, *Tiferet* is associated with the color green, and thus trees and plants are considered a beautiful expression of *Tiferet*. Green growing things manifest the energy of receiving as they take in sun, water, and nutrients from the soil. At the same time, they share with us oxygen, fruit, flowers, shade, shelter, and their own beauty. This giving and sharing is part of their very nature, despite the effort involved in such growth. To become tall—indeed, to break through the ground at all—trees must resist the downward pull of gravity, which kabbalists associate with the desire to receive for the self alone—the wish for short-term gratification, the desire to take the easy way out. Yet despite this powerful force, trees grow upward, creating long, healthy lives and giving as they grow.

Because *Tiferet* is such a healing energy, I often suggest to patients that they meditate on trees. If you'd like more healing *Tiferet* energy in your life, practice this meditation. It works best if you can spend some time experiencing the energy of an actual tree, but you can also achieve powerful effects simply by visualizing a tree.

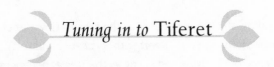

Tuning in to Tiferet

PREPARATION

1. Place yourself under a tree—or see a tree in your mind's eye. Sit in a comfortable position with your hands resting loosely in your lap. Don't fold your hands or cross your feet—allow the right and left parts of your body to remain separate.

2. Close your eyes and take 10 deep, slow breaths. Don't force your breath but rather allow it to float gently, in and out.

3. Open your eyes and observe the tree—or, in your mind's eye, bring into focus the image of a tree.

MEDITATION

1. Allow yourself to focus on the experience of this tree. Think of yourself as becoming one with the tree, feeling what it feels. Experience the sap rising from your roots, up from the depths of the earth and into your topmost branches. Feel the effort of the sap to push upward, against the force of gravity. Experience the gentle opening of your leaves as they absorb the sun and moisture in the air, as the nourishment of the sap flows into them. As you breathe out, notice the healing oxygen that each leaf is sharing with the world. Experience your sheltering branches, spread wide to protect the creatures below from sun and rain. Allow the scents and sights and sensations of the tree to penetrate your body as you become one with the tree.

2. Now connect to your own *Sefira* of *Tiferet,* the vessel of energy that surrounds your heart. What color is this *Sefira?* How large is it? What quality does the energy have—glowing? Pulsing? Shining serenely? Do you sense an imbalance here, an excess of energy, a blockage or a lack? Without judgment or opinion, experience your own *Tiferet.*

3. Finally, allow the healing energy of the tree to flow directly into your heart, infusing your *Tiferet* with its beauty and splendor. Feel the balance of receiving and giving as the tree experiences it—and then feel that balance within yourself. Notice how this infusion of energy affects your own *Tiferet*—how it affects the color, size, shape, and quality of your own heart vessel. Breathe for a few moments with the tree, your two energies connected. Remind yourself that this is a feeling that you can recapture whenever you want to, simply by remembering this moment.

NETZACH AND *HOD:* STRIDING FORWARD INTO LIFE

The famous scholar Rabbi Pinchas was known for his charismatic personality, which attracted to him numerous townspeople seeking from him advice, blessings, and the solutions to their daily problems. The rabbi appreciated his followers, but he felt that his own time for studying the Torah was being eaten away by the continual demands on his time. One day he prayed, "Dear God, let people shun me, so that I have the time for prayer and study that I require."

Sure enough, the next day, even though Rabbi Pinchas stood as usual at his window, not a single passerby paused to greet him. He spent the morning engrossed in prayer, enjoying the unusual quiet. His solitude continued even through the lunch hour, when for once no follower came to join him or to enjoy his well-known hospitality.

Then Rabbi Pinchas's wife returned home from the market and reported a strange thing: not a single person had greeted her or even spoken to her, though she had greeted many in her usual friendly way.

"This must be God's response to my prayer, which evidently extends to my entire household," Rabbi Pinchas explained. His wife began to cry at the thought of such isolation, though of course she supported her husband's study.

Then it was time for Succos, the Jewish festival in which every household is supposed to build a *succah*, a little shed decorated with fruits and flowers. Rabbi Pinchas usually had more help than he needed to build his *succah*, but this year, he was forced to do it alone.

Finally, though, the *succah* was complete, and Rabbi Pinchas invited the spirits of the patriarchs to join him inside, as he always did. This year, however, the patriarch Abraham refused to enter the rabbi's *succah*. "How can I come into a place," he asked, "where none of my children is welcome?" Thus did Rabbi Pinchas recognize his error. He prayed to God to be free of the spell, and once again, his home was full of followers and friends, all seeking to share their burdens with the rabbi and to receive his insight into their daily lives.

—ADAPTED WITH PERMISSION FROM *NOT JUST STORIES*,
RABBI ABRAHAM J. TWERSKI, M.D.,
ARTSCROLL/MESORAH PUBLICATIONS

Rabbi Pinchas was struggling with a problem familiar to many of us: balancing our wish to stride forward into the very midst of life with our occasional need to retreat into solitude. The *Sefira* located at our right hip, *Netzach*—victory, endurance— represents the wish to move forward and engage with others, while *Hod,* at our left hip—majesty—is the still, calm energy that allows others to come to us.

In kabbalistic tradition, *Netzach* embodies the energy of Moses, the powerful orator who went forth to engage in battle with the Pharaoh, mobilized the Jewish people, and encouraged them to leave Egypt. *Hod,* on the other hand, is associated with Aaron, Moses's brother, a quiet, shy man who stuttered when he spoke, but who was reputed to have the gift of prophecy and who was a far more approachable figure than the mighty Moses. Moses represented God's victory in the world, but Aaron helped translate that victory into accessible terms.

I often think of the *Netzach–Hod* duality when dealing with my patients. Sometimes they require me to speak clearly and persuasively, to challenge them, to point out decisions that might be unhealthy for them even as I urge them to make healthier choices. This is *Netzach* energy, and while I don't believe I have the kind of magnetism and charisma evinced by Moses—or even by Rabbi Pinchas—I do sometimes see my role in similar terms.

Other times, however, *Hod* energy is more appropriate for healing—that quiet empathy where I simply sit and listen, allowing my patients to express their worries, concerns, wishes, and fears. Such a role may not be charismatic or glamorous, but it may be precisely what is needed in the healing process.

Like Rabbi Pinchas, I find myself torn between my wish to be out in the world—working with patients, taking new courses in Kabbalah—and my desire to be home alone, engaged in study and solitude, replenishing my spirit. I've come to see that *Netzach* without *Hod* can easily become a kind of egotistical display, an empty exercise of charisma for the sake of amassing power. Yet, as Rabbi Pinchas discovered, *Hod* without *Netzach* can become another kind of selfishness, in which solitude isolates us from our community and its concerns. As in all things, our goal must be to find a kind of balance between the leg that strides forward with victorious movement and the leg that rests in majestic stillness.

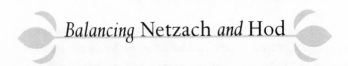

Balancing Netzach *and* Hod

PREPARATION

1. Choose a pleasant site for a walk that includes a peaceful place to rest. You might practice this meditation in a natural setting—the woods, the beach, a quiet country road—or you might select a city or suburban neighborhood that you enjoy. Just find a location where you enjoy both moving and sitting still, and allow yourself 15 to 30 minutes.

2. Remember not to cross your arms or hands during the exercise, and when you come to a resting position, don't cross your legs or feet. As always, allow the right and left parts of your body to remain separate.

3. Before you begin, prepare yourself by closing your eyes for a moment and taking a few slow breaths. With each breath, clear your mind, so that your awareness is free to be completely absorbed in the meditation you are about to begin.

MEDITATION

1. Open your eyes and begin to walk. Allow yourself to become completely aware of the sensation of moving forward into the world. Feel each hip as your legs stride forward and are pushed back. Notice the way your knees bend to allow your stride to be springy and loose. Focus for a moment on your flexible ankles, your strong feet, the way your soles land on the ground and push off from it again. Become aware of your arms, dangling loosely by your side or perhaps swinging slightly to match your stride. Notice your spine, rising up out of your hips, and the way your neck helps your head balance lightly at the top of your body. Feel your eyes looking forward as you move forward. Become aware of every detail of moving forward through space.

2. After you have been walking for a while—perhaps 5 minutes or so—find a place to come to a halt. You might simply stand in space, not moving, or you might want to lean, perch, or sit somewhere. Whatever you choose, come to a complete stop.

3. Pay attention. Notice every aspect of your body, in stillness now as it was in movement before. Become aware of how your legs feel when they are at rest—how your hips fit into your pelvis, how your legs extend downward from your hips. How do your knees feel? Focus on your ankles, your toes, the soles of your feet. Become

aware of your spine, your back, your neck, your head. Experience stillness as fully as you can.

4. After about 5 minutes, push off again. Now become fully aware of moving, just as a moment ago you were fully aware of being still. What new aspects of moving forward do you notice, now that you have been still for a while? What new sensations can you discover in your hips, your legs, your feet, your spine, your head? How does the world look to you now? How do you feel as you move?

5. Gradually, bring your awareness to *Netzach,* the *Sefira* located over your right hip. See this *Sefira* as clearly as you can—its color, size, shape, and quality. Without judgment or opinions, notice if this energy is flowing or blocked. Become aware of any excesses or lacks. Ask yourself, "What could I do in my life to get my *Netzach* energy flowing?" and notice what answers come to mind.

6. Come once again to rest, and visualize *Hod,* the *Sefira* located over your left hip. Again, see this *Sefira* as clearly as you can—its color, size, shape, and quality. Without judgment or opinions, notice if this energy is flowing or blocked. Become aware of any excesses or lacks. Ask yourself, "What could I do in my life to get my *Hod* energy flowing?" and notice what answers come to mind.

7. When you are ready, begin to move again—more slowly this time. Try as you move to notice the balance of movement and stillness that is in every movement. Pause for a moment and stand still. Can you feel yourself still moving, even as your body remains at rest? All of life is a balance of movement and stillness, and both energies are always within us, all the time. Find the balance of *Netzach* and *Hod* within yourself, whether you are moving or still. Then remind yourself that whenever you feel "out of balance," you can simply visualize this image once again—and instantly, your balance can be restored.

YESOD: CREATING A STRONG FOUNDATION

> As the whirlwind passeth, so is the wicked no more: but the
> righteous is an everlasting foundation.
>
> —PROVERBS 10:25

The central-column *Sefira* located over the groin is known as *Yesod,* which means "foundation." *Yesod* is considered the foundation of all life on earth—literally, because of the generative power of the male sexual organ, with which this *Sefira* is associated, but also figuratively, in the sense that *Yesod* is the funnel through which all of the upper *Sefirot* may flow. *Chochma, Bina,* and *Da'at,* which express the mind, and *Chesed, Gevurah, Tiferet, Hod,* and *Netzach,* which express emotion, all flow through *Yesod*—intention. Therefore, a strong *Yesod* energy allows us to forcefully communicate our intentions and manifest them in the world, often even without speaking.

In his book *Practical Kabbalah,* Rabbi Laibl Wolf associates *Yesod* with the kabbalistic notion of *kavannah,* "intention," particularly the intention to communicate. Parents and children manifest their intentions to one another without speech, Rabbi Wolf points out. He also cites some fascinating experiments conducted by Jacobo Grinberg-Zylberbaum's research team at the Universidad National Autonoma de Mexico. In these studies, researchers found that various subjects, separated by considerable distance, nevertheless manifested strong correlations between brain-wave patterns, as measured by electroencephalograms (EEG)—but only when the subjects intended to focus on one another. The intention to communicate is apparently so powerful that it can transcend long distances and can occur without speech. This is the energy of *Yesod.*

Although *Yesod* is traditionally associated with the penis, both men and women manifest *Yesod* energy, just as both sexes possess *Malchut,* the female receptive energy generated by the tenth *Sefira,* located at the soles of the feet. Just as the other *Sefirot* must be balanced and harmonized, so is it important to balance *Yesod* and *Malchut*—the active ability to put our intentions out into the world, and the receptive power to "go with the flow."

MALCHUT—BRINGING OUR INTENTIONS INTO THE WORLD

I am the rose of Sharon, and the lily of the valleys.

As the lily among thorns, so is my love among the daughters.

—SONG OF SOLOMON 2:1, 2

The Song of Solomon is considered by kabbalists and Torah scholars to be the holiest book of the Bible, for its powerful verses express the longing for unity of the male and female aspects of the soul. As we have seen, *Yesod* represents the male aspects of our nature, while *Malchut* expresses our female side.

In Kabbalah, *Malchut* has two nicknames. One is the *Imma Tata'ah,* the "Lower Mother." If *Bina* is the higher mother, nourishing divine inspiration and translating it into earthly form, *Malchut* is the lower mother, who helps manifest the other *Sefirot,* translating the emotions of *Chesed, Gevurah, Tiferet, Hod,* and *Netzach* and the intentionality of *Yesod* into concrete action.

Malchut is also known as *Alma D'Itgalya,* or "the Revealed World." Whereas *Bina* is considered "the hidden world"—the site of potential behavior—*Malchut* is the energy that brings our behavior into the light.

Some kabbalistic traditions consider *Malchut* to be located at the soles of the feet, representing the point of connection between humans and the earth. Other traditions associate *Malchut* with the mouth, the part of the body that speaks and reveals what is inside.

The literal translation of *Malchut* is "sovereignty," based on the Hebrew word *melech*, or "king." Because the energies of all the other *Sefirot* flow into the nurturing vessels of *Malchut*, the Creator's sovereignty is manifested in this vessel.

A HEALING INTIMACY WITH THE *SEFIROT*

> It only takes a little courage to fulfill wishes which until then had been regarded as unattainable.
>
> —SIGMUND FREUD

When Angelita returned after thirty days, I could see at a glance that she was doing better than the last time I had seen her. Although she had had one or two headaches during the previous month, she felt her condition was improving, and she was confident that it would continue to improve.

More important, though, I could see that she had a softer, more relaxed look about her. She told me that on one of her "required" 10-minute walks, she had passed a community garden, a large vacant lot where a number of her neighbors had their own little plots. Impulsively, she had gone into the garden and asked about getting a plot of her own. Now she was leaving work much earlier to be able to garden during the last hours of daylight, and she had begun making friends with some of her fellow gardeners. Although her journey was far from over, I could see that Angelita had begun the powerful process of bringing her *Sefirot* into balance—with profound consequences for her health and happiness.

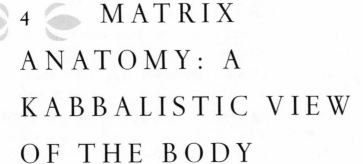

4 MATRIX ANATOMY: A KABBALISTIC VIEW OF THE BODY

THE ZOHAR—

> *Whoever labors in the Torah upholds the world as a whole, for a man's body consists of . . . parts . . . all acting and reacting upon each other, so as to form one organism. So does the world at large consist of . . . things, which when they properly act and react upon each other together form literally one organic body.*

MY patient Randolph was worried.

He had just gotten back the results of his angiogram—a cardiac test that measures the amount of blockage in the arteries—and he was now coming to terms with the news that his arteries were severely blocked. According to conventional medical wisdom, he was at high risk for a heart attack, especially since he'd already had angina—chest pain—and a cardiogram had revealed an irregular rhythm in his heart.

Normally, such a diagnosis would mean Randolph needed bypass surgery or an angioplasty, in which plaque is literally scraped out of the arteries. These are invasive and debilitating procedures, and if the underlying problem is not corrected, the patient often must return to the hospital for a second, third, or even fourth operation.

But Randolph was a hard-driving Wall Street veteran in his sixties who had never been willing to accept defeat. Right from our first meeting, he was full of ideas about what he could do to improve his health.

"I've heard about diet plans, where you reduce the amount of fat you eat," he offered. "Should I be doing that? Or maybe I'm supposed to meditate—you know, to calm myself down? Or do I have to cut back my hours at work, stop being such a Type A personality, that kind of thing?"

I smiled at his eagerness. "I'm not against any of the approaches you mentioned," I told him. "And they certainly won't do any harm. But a kabbalistic perspective is somewhat different. For that matter, modern science itself has moved beyond those particular responses."

Randolph listened intently as I explained the dual nature of Matrix Anatomy. On the one hand, we have to view the body in a holistic way, understanding that every organ affects every other organ and that our entire anatomy operates as a single interactive unit. Yet, we must also be aware that each of our organs literally has its own consciousness, its own spiritual underpinnings, its own particular needs, desires, and responses. I like to think of each organ as having its own metaphysical theme within a larger theme of the entire body. As Job said, "From my flesh do I see God."

I told Randolph that if he preferred, I could simply make some suggestions concerning diet, herbal treatments, meditation, and the like, but he quickly shook his head.

"You're telling me that every organ is important," he said. "So

I want to learn about all of them. Give me the big picture, then tell me where I fit into it. That's the way I work in business, and that's the way I want to approach my health, too."

"Well, if you're looking for the big picture," I told him, "then we have to start with the most important organ of all—the human brain."

THE HEALING BRAIN

> The brain is the throne of mercy.
>
> —THE ZOHAR

When I was still in medical school, there were two major cutting-edge fields: genetics and the brain.

A whole new body of research had begun to suggest that many disorders—including heart disease, cancer, and Alzheimer's—might be strongly influenced by our genetic heritage. Geneticists had always known that such rare conditions as sickle-cell anemia, Tay Sachs, and other congenital diseases were genetically determined, to the point where many such disorders could be associated with particular ethnic groups, such as African Americans or Ashkenazi Jews. Now, though, scientists were beginning to associate more widespread diseases with genetic programming, even suggesting that we might someday be able to identify cancer- or heart-disease-prone children in the womb.

Inspired by these discoveries, geneticists were also arguing that many personality traits, such as shyness, sensitivity, and creativity, were also genetically determined. The new interest in genetics gave rise to the Human Genome Project, in which scientists believed they had mapped every aspect of the human genetic inheritance. Finally, the geneticists promised, we would have a thorough scientific understanding of exactly what it meant to be human.

Meanwhile, a lot of new research was coming out about the brain, revealing the many ways that emotions, mental states, and thought processes could be tracked biochemically. Numerous psychological states that had once been treated with therapy—including depression, anxiety, and difficulties paying attention—were now being viewed as neurochemical imbalances and treated with medication. Whereas pioneering psychotherapists like Auschwitz survivor Viktor Frankl had seen existential despair as a spiritual problem, the new therapy revolved around diagnostic manuals and prescription pads. As far as I could see, the mechanistic view of the human body that I'd found so distressing was now being extended to the human mind and spirit, as well. The prevailing scientific view seemed to equate the mind and the brain—to imagine that every human thought, ability, or choice could ultimately be reduced to a biochemical event.

Instinctively, I resisted the idea that our free will and our creative potential are circumscribed by the physical limits of the "gray matter" within our skulls, but this is what I and my fellow physicians were taught. Geneticists and neurologists seemed to agree that we were no more than a set of biochemical elements with a limited number of predetermined possibilities. And if some of these scientists happened, in their private lives, to hold to some religious faith, they saw no relationship between that fairy-tale belief and the hard, cold world of "real science."

Imagine my surprise—and relief—when I came upon *The Healing Brain,* the pioneering 1987 work written by psychologist Robert Ornstein and physician David Sobel. Ornstein, a Stanford University professor of neurobiology, and Sobel, director of protective medicine in the Kaiser-Permanente Health System, argued that the brain's primary purpose was to heal the body, activating our immune system, alleviating pain, and regulating our physical functions in response to the external world. Far from seeing the brain as a passive biochemical entity, Ornstein and Sobel portrayed this marvelous organ as an active instrument of healing. Moreover, the authors argued, a person's beliefs, attitudes, and daily practice could have an enormous influence on the brain, perhaps even transcending genetic tendencies to heart disease, cancer, and other disorders.

Ornstein and Sobel's work was beautifully complemented, a decade later, by Candace Pert's 1999 *Molecules of Emotion: The Science Behind Mind-Body Medicine.* Pert's specialty is brain chemistry, and in 1972 she was lauded for her groundbreaking work on the brain's production of opiates and endorphins, natural painkillers and mood-regulators that alleviate sensations of physical distress. She went on to describe the ways that endorphins and opiates are sent all over the body, so that our emotions are literally experienced in our immune system, our heart, and many other organs. Suddenly the notion of "a happy immune system" or "an angry gut" was far more than a metaphor—it was an accurate biological description of how our bodies worked. (I discuss the emotional life of the gastrointestinal system in my book *Gut Reactions.*)

Pert's work inspired an even more startling discovery: emotions originate in the body as well as the brain. Apparently, the heart and other organs actually produce their own "messenger molecules," so that states of compassion, love, and appreciation actually cause the heart to redirect the brain. In response, the brain releases a different ratio of neurotransmitters, creating a new hormonal balance. Thus, when we experience love, our level of stress hormones drops, particularly cortisol—associated with weight gain, menstrual problems, and a wide variety of stress-related illnesses.

As a scientist, I found this work exciting. And when I came to study Kabbalah, I discovered a remarkable correspondence between the 2,000-year-old Zohar and the late twentieth-century work of Ornstein, Sobel, Pert, and others. The "healing brain" was truly a throne of mercy, while, as the Zohar had insisted, the brain really does listen to the commands of the heart. But according to the Zohar, the brain is the ultimate commander, and it can overrule the heart when necessary.

Indeed, I began to realize that human consciousness could change even our genetic makeup. Some studies of E. coli bacteria conducted by researchers at Albert Einstein College of Medicine revealed that genes can sense their environment and alter themselves accordingly, causing their own mutations at a rate that could not be explained by simple Darwinian evolution.

Likewise, studies conducted by Glen Rein, Ph.D., and Rollin McCraty, at the International Society for the Study of Subtle Energies and Energy Medicine, revealed the powerful effects of love. The researchers discovered that when people who were skilled at meditation focused on creating loving states within themselves, their DNA actually uncoiled further—a tremendous indicator of good health and a sign that love has a direct line of communication to the very core of life itself.

I also came across studies suggesting that meditation and hypnosis could change the production of messenger RNA. Messenger RNA is the biochemical substance used by our genes to communicate instructions to the rest of our body. These genetic studies seemed to imply that genetic expression could literally be altered by consciousness, whether that consciousness was responding to an outside force, such as hypnosis, or an internal one, like meditation.

In other words, the science I had been taught in medical school was wrong—not only from a religious viewpoint but also simply as science. The mechanistic, deterministic view of genes and the brain had been outstripped by new theories that portrayed human biology not as a limited set of chemical possibilities but rather as a malleable, responsive, and open-ended system.

THE MIND AND THE BRAIN

> This leaves us with a clear physiological fact . . . moment by moment we choose and sculpt how our ever-changing minds will work, we choose who we will be the next moment in a very real sense, and these choices are left embossed in physical form on our material selves.
>
> —MEZERNICH AND DECHARMS, CITED BY JEFFREY SCHWARTZ, M.D., AND SHARON BEGLEY, *THE MIND AND THE BRAIN: NEUROPLASTICITY AND THE POWER OF MENTAL FORCE*

The biochemists and geneticists were all doing exciting work. But it was the 2002 publication of *The Mind and the Brain* that really showed me the extent to which modern science has "caught up" with the precepts of Kabbalah.

The Mind and the Brain details the work of UCLA psychiatrist Jeffrey Schwartz, M.D., a specialist in obsessive-compulsive disorder, or OCD. Schwartz and co-author Sharon Begley, a *Wall Street Journal* science columnist, explain that OCD can be viewed as the result of faulty wiring in the brain, circuitry that literally compels OCD patients to engage in such repetitive behavior as handwashing, counting, and other elaborate rituals. Clearly, there is a biochemical basis for OCD, a physical disorder within the brain itself.

Yet Schwartz found that when his OCD patients became aware of the reasons for their behavior and learned to see themselves as "more than" their brains, they could gradually transcend their biochemical programming. In Schwartz's successful four-step program, OCD patients learned about the brain's role in their disorder. Then they were taught to make different choices, literally activating another portion of their brain that could help override the faulty messages instructing them to engage in compulsive behavior. Through the exercise of their free wills, Schwartz's patients actually reworked their own biochemistry, "generat[ing] a mental force that changes brain circuitry."

Schwartz realized that his findings were not limited to OCD patients. He has begun to have some success using his method with patients suffering from Tourette's syndrome, a compulsion that causes physical twitching and the repetition of obscene and inappropriate language. He also believes his method might be of use to patients who suffer from depression. Although he readily agrees with the prevailing scientific view that depression has a biochemical component, he believes that once depressed patients understand that they are more than their brains, they can use their minds to reprogram their faulty biochemistry, just as his OCD patients have done.

More broadly, Schwartz believes that all of us are capable of creating new abilities within our brains, whether we suffer from brain-chemistry problems or not. A skilled pianist, for example, might practice a sequence of notes over and over again. This activity helps to make her fingers more limber, but it also creates a new pathway within her brain, a pathway on which she can rely as she plays the same concerto again and again. More significantly, studies have shown that the pianist can create the exact same pathway without even playing the notes, but simply by imagining them. Apparently that mental activity rewires her brain just as efficiently as the actual physical experience of playing.

These examples are striking enough, but a Matrix Healing

approach makes it clear that we can reprogram our brains in even more dramatic ways, overcoming disease and creating health. Indeed, this seems to be what people do when they have multiple personalities. As we saw in Chapter 2, each personality has the same basic brain chemistry to work with, but it also has "a mind of its own" that molds and reshapes that brain chemistry to respond in different ways. The man who was stung by a wasp, for example, had only a single brain, with an apparently finite amount of biochemical material. Yet one of his personalities called for that brain to generate the biochemical cascade that produces a severe allergic response, even as another personality instructed the same brain to alter its biochemistry and eliminate all allergic symptoms.

Schwartz points out that every one of his OCD patients started out with a defective brain—a brain whose faulty chemistry, left to its own devices, drove each patient to engage in apparently uncontrollable unwanted behavior. Yet his patients were also larger than their brains, and their minds were able to instruct their brains in new ways. Contrary to the prevailing wisdom in contemporary neuroscience, Schwartz concluded that our minds are indeed greater than our brains.

To describe what he meant by "mind," Schwartz drew on the quantum physics notion of an *emergent phenomenon:* "one whose characteristics or behaviors cannot be explained in terms of the sum of its parts. . . ." In other words, Schwartz argued, we are a whole that is larger than the sum of our brain's parts. That larger whole is something that he called mind, that physical but not only physical entity that "cannot be wholly explained by brain."

As a Matrix Healer, I like Schwartz's theories very much because they offer a scientific basis for what Kabbalah has been saying for a long time: we are our bodies, yes, but we are also more than our bodies. As we saw in Chapter 3, the Light that moves through the ten *Sefirot* is both physical and something more, even as the *Sefirot* themselves are multidimensional: physical, emotional, and spiritual all at the same time.

Moreover, the mind is not found only in the brain. As Pert's theories suggest—and as the notion of *Sefirot* supports—there is a kind of intelligence that exists throughout our bodies, so that heart, liver, lungs, and other organs each possess its own special knowledge. Such knowledge may be synthesized in the brain, but it cannot be limited to that physical portion of ourselves. Our entire body has its own intelligence, which Schwartz calls *mind,* and which Matrix Healing calls our *proactive natures*—our ability to be like the Creator.

FIRE AND WATER: NEW THEORIES OF INFLAMMATION

Disease is the fire that consumes the body.

—THE ZOHAR

This vivid imagery from the 2,000-year-old Zohar anticipates one of the latest scientific discoveries: that many diseases—including heart disease, cancer, osteoporosis, arthritis, asthma, and Alzheimer's—are related to inflammation. Although modern science has lost much of the Zohar's poetry, it's not much of a stretch to see inflammation as a kind of anatomical fire.

Ironically, inflammation is the body's healing response to infection, irritation, or injury. Blood rushes to the distressed site, bringing its nutrients (plasma) and white blood cells (leukocytes). These white blood cells are a crucial part of the body's immune system, designed to devour offending cells and foreign bodies, to kill off invading hosts, and to help carry away dead tissue. White blood cells are somewhat larger than the usual nutrients carried by the capillaries, the tiniest blood vessels, so the capillaries retract their endothelial cells, weakening their walls to allow these larger molecules to wash through.

This response to inflammation produces a number of well-known symptoms:

- Redness, from the swelling of the small blood vessels.

- Heat—an increase in temperature, from the increased blood flow and from the fever induced by some of the body's immune response.

- Swelling, from the accumulation of fluid and the inflammatory cells themselves.

- Pain, from the stretching and distortion of the tissues, swollen by excess blood, white blood cells, and in some cases, pus, a combination of excess liquid and dead tissue. Some of the body's chemical responses to infection and injury—the hormones known as bradykinin, the prostaglandins, and serotonin—are also known to induce pain.

The irony continues throughout the healing process, for the very inflammation that helps to heal us can also make us sick. On an immediate level, we're all familiar with the redness, swelling, heat, and pain that come with a scraped knee, a minor infection, or even a too-well-scratched mosquito bite. But when inflammation takes place within our bodies, it can have more serious long-term consequences. Asthma and other severe allergic reactions, for example, are now understood to be mistaken autoimmune responses. The body encounters something that is in fact harmless—pollen, some kind of nontoxic food, or the fluid from a bee sting—and reacts as though the foreign substance represents mortal danger. The immune response—heat, swelling, and a flood of white blood cells—is not really necessary, but the body "thinks" it is. And ironically, it is the immune response—not the foreign substance—that endangers the patient. In asthma, the lungs become so inflamed that the airways swell shut and the patient cannot breathe. A severe allergic reaction can produce a similar effect—the lungs swell shut, or perhaps massive swelling and inflammation occur at the site of a bee sting. In both cases, the body is responding to the inflammation caused by its own (mistaken and exaggerated) immune response.

According to pioneering new studies, inflammation can also lead to heart disease. As with asthma and allergies, "the body's defense mechanism turns into a betrayal," according to an October 7, 1999, *Wall Street Journal* article by Ron Winslow, quoting Valentin Fuster, director of cardiovascular research at Mount Sinai School of Medicine, in New York City. The article also quotes Peter Libby, chief of cardiovascular medicine at Harvard Medical School and Brigham and Women's Hospital, who says, "There is an inflammatory response that alters the biology of the artery wall. . . . [In the process] the normal defense mechanisms get turned against you."

According to this research, heart disease may begin with an initial irritation that takes place as early as adolescence. This irritation might be caused by infection, cigarette smoke, or various toxins in the blood that have not been properly filtered out by the liver. The body's immune system responds to the irritation, causing inflammation. This inflammation in turn can damage the arterial walls.

Of course, if the initial irritation is brief and temporary, the inflammation recedes and there's no problem. Heart disease occurs, however, when the artery walls are repeatedly exposed to irritation—from chronic or repeated infections; from cigarette smoke or other toxins in the blood; from high cholesterol, which thickens the blood and causes it to scrape against the arterial walls; and/or from plaque, pockets of excess fat that build up within the arteries. A diet high in sugar and/or white flour can also irritate the arterial walls, increasing the risk of heart disease.

If these conditions exist, what Dr. Libby calls "a smoldering process" begins. A vicious cycle of infection and irritation, on the one hand, and immune-system-induced inflammation, on the other, weakens the arterial walls. Deposits of plaque are also contained in walls of tissue—walls that are likewise weakened by inflammation. If these walls rupture, the plaque is released, creating a sudden massive clot that can block an artery and cause a heart attack.

Of course, inflammation is supposed to help clear plaque, which the body properly reads as a foreign substance that is blocking the artery and needs to be removed. But the immune system is not equipped to cope with too much plaque or with plaque that is too fatty. In such cases, the immune system becomes overwhelmed. Although immune cells try to remove the fat by eating it, they become engorged with fat and die. These dead cells then become part of the mass of plaque, which grows larger and larger, waiting to respond to a heart-attack trigger— stress, exertion, or another infection.

When I explained this process to my patient Randolph, he immediately assumed that high levels of cholesterol and a high degree of arterial blockage present the highest levels of risk. That's what we used to think, but recent research shows that it isn't true. Many patients with high cholesterol never experience a heart attack, while some patients with relatively low cholesterol do. Likewise, an angiogram might pick up on huge plaque deposits that are not in particular danger of rupture, while missing smaller, more unstable plaque deposits that will in fact rupture.

Therefore, I told Randolph, we are now coming to believe that the more reliable indicators of cardiac risk are various markers of inflammation, including a substance called c-reactive protein. It's not the amount of fat that's the problem but, rather, the degree of inflammation. In other words, rather than simply focusing on cholesterol levels or arterial blockage, we need to look at the "fire in the body" described in the Zohar.

THE HEART AND THE LIVER

> It is bile that consumes the arteries and ultimately all the organs.
>
> —THE ZOHAR

The Zohar and modern medical opinion agree: to properly understand heart disease, we can't stop with the heart or even with the circulatory system—we have to go on to the liver, the producer of bile and the site of toxins and free radicals.

The liver's job is to purify toxins from the blood. Anything impure or indigestible in our food gets filtered out by the liver, which is also charged with detoxifying the poisons from alcohol, cigarette smoke, recreational drugs, prescription medications, additives, preservatives, pollution, toxic fumes, and an excess of processed sugar. The liver is also responsible for metabolizing fat and turning it into various types of cholesterol.

For most of human history, people had relatively low-fat diets, consumed only natural foods, avoided tobacco, and used alcohol and drugs only on ceremonial occasions. In those days, the liver had a relatively easy job. In our modern society, however, virtually everything we eat, drink, and breathe contains some ingredient that stresses the liver. Because the liver is also charged with clearing excess estrogen from the body, women with overstressed livers are vulnerable to osteoporosis, weight gain, and problems with menstrual cycles and menopause. And all of us are subject to the inflammation that can result from toxins in the blood.

Remember, our liver's job is to metabolize fat and remove toxins from the bloodstream, so that they can be discharged through urination. When our livers aren't working efficiently—overstressed by excess fat, sugar, pollution, medications, and additives—too many toxins remain in our bloodstream, causing inflammation and helping to create the free radicals that lead to disease and aging. Excess toxins also tend to spill over into the bile, giving rise to the Zohar's comment.

So far, we're entirely in the territory of medical science. But in Matrix Healing, we understand that every part of the human body has an emotional and spiritual dimension as well as a physical one. In Kabbalah, the liver—and a related organ, the spleen—are the seat of reactive emotions. The liver is the seat of anger, jealousy, and hatred, while the spleen is the site of fear, anxiety, and doubt. This emotional anatomy shows us that there's a relationship between a weakened, toxic liver and reactive responses. Whenever we greet a life situation with anger, jealousy, or hatred, we impair our liver's ability to detoxify our blood. Whenever we respond with fear, anxiety, or doubt, we weaken our spleen, which in turn weakens our liver.

Of course, medical science has also caught up with Matrix Healing here, at least to some extent. These reactive emotions—lumped in a general way under the heading of "stress"—are well known to cause problems for our bodies, and have been related to heart disease, cancer, ulcers, colitis, migraine, and a host of other inflammatory diseases. From a kabbalistic perspective, however, it's not simply stress—a challenge to the body—that creates the problem. It's *reactivity*—responding as weak and passive beings, rather than as powerful, creative Vessels of the Light. Thus, our health does not require us to avoid stress, but only to avoid reactive responses to stress. When we can replace reactive responses with proactive choices, meeting life's challenges with serenity and joy, we strengthen our livers, reduce the number of free radicals within our system, and decrease the inflammatory responses that lead to heart disease, cancer, asthma, and other diseases.

When I explained this to Randolph, he became very excited. Having read about Type A personalities and the role of stress in heart disease, he had worried that caring for his health meant withdrawing from his high-pressure job and choosing a more peaceful existence, which he sardonically referred to as "a boring little house in the country." He loved his work, though, and he was overjoyed to realize that he didn't have to leave his job or even necessarily cut back his hours. Rather, he had to change his attitude toward his work and the stresses it created.

I told Randolph that changing his diet would almost certainly improve the health of his heart. Cutting back on hydrogenated and saturated fats would relieve the stress on his liver, as would giving up processed sugar. In kabbalistic terms, I told him, consuming processed sugar represents Receiving for the Self Alone, so it's no wonder that too much sugar raises levels of triglycerides—fats—in the blood and increases the risk of heart disease. (For more on food choices and their meaning, see the next chapter.)

I also suggested that Randolph consider taking such herbal supplements as green tea, which works to quench free radicals and decrease fibrinogen levels, and octicosanol, which reduces "bad" cholesterol, increases "good" cholesterol, and lowers blood pressure. What was exciting to both of us, however, was the way these nutritional suggestions took on a new meaning in the larger context of Matrix Anatomy. Now that Randolph understood how his body worked and saw the larger spiritual meaning of the various organs, he was eager to support proactive choices and to avoid reactive behavior. He wasn't mechanistically cutting the fats out of his diet or fearfully avoiding sugar. Instead, he saw himself as lovingly supporting his organs, enabling them to do the job they were meant to do, while bringing himself greater emotional and spiritual satisfaction. He did, in fact, follow many of the traditional prescriptions of a "heart-healthy" diet—but in a way that flowed from his deeper understanding. In my view, this attitude toward herbal supplements and diet means far more than the ingredients themselves. We doctors already know that a treatment may work beautifully with one patient and have very little impact on the next. I believe that this difference in effectiveness is due mainly to the larger spiritual context in which the treatment takes place. By seeing his body in terms of Matrix Anatomy, Randolph became an active participant in his own healing—and his health improved accordingly.

Indeed, the following year, Randolph's angiogram revealed that the blockage in his arteries had decreased slightly. Although a more dramatic change would have been nice, perhaps it was just that tiny shift that made the difference between getting and not getting a heart attack. And when I measured Randolph's c-reactive proteins—the measure of inflammation that has been shown to be a remarkable indicator of cardiac risk—I was pleased to find that they had actually decreased. Through a combination of nutritional, spiritual, and emotional changes, Randolph had lowered the inflammation within his body and significantly decreased his risk of heart attack. These are the kinds of triumphs that Matrix Healing makes possible—an integration of physical, mental, and spiritual healing.

THE COOLING BREATH OF THE LUNGS

> The heart burns so hot that without the cooling breath of the lungs, it would burn up not only itself, but the whole world.
>
> —THE ZOHAR

Among the practices that Randolph found most helpful were the breathing exercises I taught him. He liked the kabbalistic image that the cool breath of the lungs was needed to cool down the hot passions of the heart, and he cherished the Zohar's description of the lungs as the wings of a dove—the bird of peace—coated in silver. Indeed, as Randolph discovered, the lungs bring peace to the body by reminding us that mercy and serenity are only a breath away. They are the expression of how we share the entire world with one another, breathing and expiring each other's air.

In kabbalistic terms, moreover, the heart and liver are associated with the color red and are considered to be part of the left column—the Desire to Receive. The heart in this imagery represents the hot, passionate wish to possess—love, power, or any other "heart's desire." The liver, as we've seen, is the seat of reactive emotions—quick, impulsive, and often selfish reactions.

The lungs, on the other hand, are associated with the color white and the central column—the Desire to Receive for the Sake of Sharing. Indeed, the very in-and-out motion of the human breath evokes the interconnectedness of receiving in order to share—sharing because one has just received.

Another way of thinking about the heart and lungs is to imagine the heart as red with confidence, pleasure, and certainty of its own power. But, as the Zohar also says, "The only whole heart is a broken heart." Lungs, which carry tiny droplets of water and which are often associated with tears and grief, are needed to cool the hot passions of the heart by bringing a measure of sorrow to counteract the heart's quick and insistent desires. Recalling the tearful griefs of others—the sorrows we inevitably feel whenever we connect to the other members of our world—is an important balance for the heart's heat.

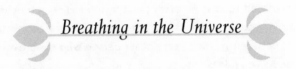

Breathing in the Universe

PREPARATION

Choose a peaceful, protected environment if you can. If you're trying these exercises at the office, close your door. If you're trying these exercises on a bus or subway, make sure you have put all your possessions out of harm's way and leave yourself enough time to make your stop. The goal is to allow your entire concentration to focus on your breathing, rather than dividing it between breathing and some other task. Remember, too, that whenever you breathe, you are always participating in the Creator's initial creation of the universe.

MEDITATION

1. Close your eyes. Close your mouth and breathe through your nose. Pull in a deep draft of air through both nostrils, allowing the breath to reach the pit of your stomach. Don't force anything . . . simply

allow the breath to float in, reaching deeper and deeper inside you. Then allow the breath to float out, until you have completely released all the air you just took in.

2. Breathe in again. Follow the air as it is drawn down through your nose, the back of your throat, your lungs, your diaphragm. Notice every moment of your breath's journey. Use your breath to unlock your awareness of your body.

3. Breathe out. Follow the air as it rises from your diaphragm, through your lungs, into your throat, up your nose, and out your two nostrils. Notice every moment of your breath's journey. Use your breath to unlock your awareness of your body.

4. Now, as you breathe, begin to visualize the air you are breathing in. Allow yourself to imagine every person who has been touched by that air. As you draw the air into your lungs, feel the connection it creates between you and every other person who has breathed that air. As you release the air from your lungs, see all the people whom the air will reach.

5. Continue to be aware of your own body. See if you can expand that awareness—without losing it—to include an awareness of the world that you touch with every breath in, every breath out. Feel the way your body is part of all the others who have breathed this air in. Feel the way your body is part of all the others who have breathed this air out. Allow your breathing to connect you to every human being in the world, all of whom have been touched by this air. Allow your breathing to connect you to every human being in the world, all of whom will be touched by this air.

6. As you finish this exercise, hold the breath in your lungs for an extra moment. Feel this as your closest connection to all the humans who have ever breathed this air, who will ever breathe this air, from the beginning of human history right up to the present

moment and on into the future. Feel how your body is a part of their bodies, how their energy and spirit are a part of your energy and spirit. Hold the breath for as long as you can, savoring this connection. Then release the breath—slowly and gently—and open your eyes.

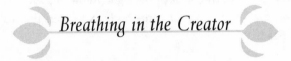

Breathing in the Creator

PREPARATION

Use the same preparation as for the previous exercise.

MEDITATION

1. Close your eyes. Close your mouth so that you can breathe through your nose. Throughout the exercise, as you draw in and release breath, do not force your breath in or push it out. Think of yourself as allowing the breath to flow through you. Visualize yourself as opening fully to the breath. Your role is to be relaxed and open, so that the breath can flow naturally through you.

2. Begin to breathe through your nostrils. As you draw the breath into your body, feel it rising through your nose into your brain. Release the breath fully, making even more room for the next breath to enter and fill your brain. Continue to breathe in and out, opening yourself to greater awareness of your body. Follow the breath as it enters your nostrils, moves through your nose, and rises into your brain . . . and then follow the breath as it falls gently from your brain and is released through your nose and out of your two nostrils. Allow your entire body to relax as your breath enters . . . and leaves . . . enters . . . and leaves.

3. When you are completely relaxed and open to the fullness of the breath as it enters and leaves your body, allow your awareness to float up to the crown of your head. Feel the crown of your head opening wider and wider with each breath ... opening to the divine Light of the universe, opening to the Light of the Creator. See the Light entering your body through the crown of your head. Allow yourself to see what color it is—white? Golden? Another color? Open yourself to the color of the Light. Allow this white or colored Light to flood your entire body as it enters the crown of your head.

4. Continue to breathe. Continue to allow your breath to float in and out through your nostrils, into your brain, up to the crown of your head. Continue to allow the Light from above to flow into your body through the crown of your head. Feel the Light flooding through your head, your throat, your lungs, your heart, your diaphragm. Feel how the Light brings its color and warmth into your body. Feel how the Light brings the abundant love of the Creator into your body. Feel how the Light—and each breath you take and each breath you release—connects you to this divine love. Feel how this Light, this love, is available to you with every single breath.

5. Now feel your own love, which starts deep within your body, in your diaphragm and in your heart, at the base of your lungs. Feel your own love rising through your lungs, your throat, your nose, and flowing out through your nostrils, and through the crown of your head, connecting you to the Creator's divine Light. Continue to breathe, feeling the flow of love, back and forth, through your lungs and nose, through the crown of your head, connecting you to the Creator, connecting the Creator to you.

6. As you complete the exercise, hold the last breath—gently—for as long as you can. As you hold this final, large breath, feel the fullness of the Creator's love within you, feel the fullness of your

love for the Creator and for the world that surrounds you. Feel
how you are a part of the Creator, a part of the world. Feel how
the love between you, the world, and the Creator continually flows
back and forth . . . and release your final breath. Open your eyes. Sit
for a moment, allowing yourself to re-create your awareness of the
flow of love, the flow of Light, as you continue to breathe.

 Breathing Through Restriction

PREPARATION

Use the same preparation as for the previous exercise.

MEDITATION

1. Close your eyes. Close your mouth so that you can breathe through
   your nose. Throughout the exercise, as you draw in and release
   breath, do not force your breath in or push it out. Think of yourself
   as allowing the breath to flow through you. Visualize yourself as
   opening fully to the breath. Your role is to be relaxed and open, so
   that the breath can flow naturally through you.

2. Keeping your shoulders relaxed and loose, expel the remaining
   breath from your body. Notice how your diaphragm contracts as
   you expel the breath. Think of yourself as giving this exhaled
   breath to the universe, even as you make room for a new breath
   within yourself.

3. Now breathe in. Notice how your diaphragm expands . . . and
   expands . . . and expands to make room for the ever-increasing
   breath. If you cannot breathe very deeply at first, start by breathing
   in on a count of two . . . then four . . . then six, eight, ten, and finally

twelve. Notice how large and expansive your diaphragm becomes as you breathe so deeply. Notice how your chest cavity expands as your lungs fill up. Notice how large you are, how much you are capable of receiving.

4. Hold this large breath as long as you can—until finally you are forced to expel it. Think of how so much receiving means that you simply *have* to share! Continue to breathe in and out, allowing yourself to fully experience the sensation of filling up—and then needing to share.

5. Now visualize each deep breath as a huge infusion of Light. Experience yourself breathing in the Light, holding it within yourself, and then returning it to the universe. Notice how the Light is temporarily restricted by your diaphragm on its way in and out—a restriction that allows you to expand to ever-greater size.

6. Finally, open your eyes as you continue to breathe. Remain aware of the sensation of your breath—pushing against the restriction of your diaphragm, expanding your chest and stomach, and then returning to the universe from whence it came. Look around you and allow your breath to connect you to everything you see. As you get up and return to your daily tasks, maintain this spirit of connectedness through an awareness of your breath.

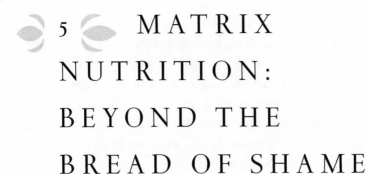

5 MATRIX NUTRITION: BEYOND THE BREAD OF SHAME

EXODUS 24:11–

And they thought of God, and they ate, and they drank.

ELEANOR was a tall, somewhat heavy woman in her mid-thirties who had had Type 2 diabetes for the past fifteen years. At our first appointment, she told me that she felt she'd been in a lifelong battle with food, struggling to keep her blood sugars down even as she desperately tried to limit her weight.

"Sometimes, frankly, I hate the idea that I have to eat in order to live," she said in a discouraged, angry tone. "I wish there were some pill I could take that would mean I didn't need to eat, or some injection you could give me that would stop me from being hungry. I'm just so tired of thinking about every bite I put into my mouth."

It's crucial for people with diabetes to be careful about what they eat, so I was glad to see that Eleanor was so committed to keeping her blood sugars at a healthy level. Although diabetics face special concerns with blood sugar, a growing body of research suggests that blood sugar levels that are too high or that fluctuate wildly can cause problems for nondiabetics as well, including cravings for sweets, weight gain, allergies, insomnia and other sleep disorders, depression, fatigue, nervousness, memory problems, inability to concentrate, "foggy thinking," and headaches—the same kinds of problems that Angelita had experienced from her high-sugar bedtime snacks, as we saw in Chapter 3.

Moreover, high or fluctuating blood-sugar levels frequently result from excessive consumption of sugar, refined carbohydrates, and the wrong kinds of fat—a diet that has also been associated with osteoporosis, heart disease, and cancer. The problems Eleanor faced with her diet were particularly urgent for people with diabetes, but they were certainly significant for many of my other patients, as well. Indeed, it was to address just such problems that I developed the Bio-Ecological Diet, an approach to food that I've shared in my book *Gut Reactions.*

There were some dietary shifts that I thought might help Eleanor to feel less hungry and more physically satisfied with the food she ate. I suggested that she eat more greens (kale, collards, chard) and green herbs (fresh dill, coriander, sage, mint); use cinnamon in her cooking to stimulate insulin production; drink eight to twelve glasses of water each day, with fresh lemon if possible; and limit her intake of carbohydrates, especially at dinner.

But I didn't think Eleanor needed help with food choices as much as a new perspective on food altogether. I was sorry to hear how distressing the whole issue of food had become for her, and I was sure that her perspective was affecting her metabolism and her digestion, as well as her mood. The attitudes and feelings we bring to the table literally affect how our bodies process the food we eat, with crucial effects on our weight, intestinal health, and ability to absorb the nutrients we ingest.

I thought that if Eleanor were able to adopt a kabbalistic vision of food, she might develop a new relationship both to food itself and to her body's need for food—a whole new understanding and appreciation of food and of life itself. I was sure that this shift in perspective would have profoundly beneficial effects on her metabolism—and, even more important, that it might actually enable her to enjoy her physical self, taking pleasure in the food she ate and in her body's response to it.

FOOD AND THE FLOW OF LIFE

> Food is a love note from God. Its letters are written by the rays of the sun. It says I love you and I shall take care of you and sustain you with the offerings of my earth. If we take time to read the love letter, by chewing carefully and feeling the messages that are stored in food by the sun, earth, wind, water, and even by those who have grown, harvested, and prepared the food, its assimilation takes on a whole new meaning. This is a specific way of receiving God's grace, a holy sacrament to be experienced slowly, carefully, and consciously.
>
> —GABRIEL COUSENS, M.D., *CONSCIOUS EATING*

The first step in understanding food from a kabbalistic perspective is to see our consumption and digestion as part of our relationship with the Creator, another instance of the interaction between Light and Vessel. After all, we must eat to live—and fortunately, nature has provided us with abundant sources of nourishment that can delight every one of our senses as well as supplying us with energy, sustaining our health, and assuring our very existence. Each time we put food into our mouths, we have the opportunity to experience the profound generosity of the universe, which has provided us with the sustenance we need in such a wonderful variety of forms. This joy in the universe's bounty has prompted the traditional Hebrew prayer that is supposed to be recited each time food is consumed: *"Blessed are you, our God, Ruler of the Universe, who brings forth bread from the earth."*

I'm not advocating a religious approach here but, rather, a new worldview: a vision of food as an outward sign of the beneficence of God or the Essence of Life, and a call to us to give in return by sharing ourselves. For far too long, we've seen food in mechanistic terms, a soulless matter of calories and nutritional units, in which food is "burned" by our digestive systems and translated into the "fuel" we need for our "engines." No wonder this mechanistic approach has led to a world full of fast food and packaged foods high in fat and sugar, of pesticide-coated vegetables and hormone-laden meats. No wonder chickens and cows are raised in high-tech farms that box them into impossibly small cages and stalls that do not even allow them the freedom to scratch in the earth or to enjoy the sunshine, and where they are slaughtered with the same casual cruelty that marked their constricted lives. No wonder obesity, diabetes, eating disorders, acid reflux and indigestion, ulcers, colitis, female hormonal problems, and cancer are on the rise, that Americans are both overfed and malnourished, that food, weight, and body shape remain the unhappy preoccupations of so many of us. Neither our bodies nor the food that nourishes them was ever meant to be treated as a soulless object, and if we insist on maintaining that relationship to food—and to ourselves—every one of us will pay the price.

As opposed to this mechanistic view, the kabbalists see food in terms of the two basic spiritual forces in the world: the Desire to Share and the Desire to Receive. From a kabbalistic point of view, our relationship to food begins with the digestive process itself, which is initially the Desire to Receive for the Self Alone. Hunger is a powerful expression of this desire—indeed, we often use the words *hunger* and *desire* interchangeably, as an acknowledgment that our wish for food is one of the most basic desires we'll ever feel.

So our hunger begins as a selfish Desire to Receive. But what happens when we choose to see the food we crave as a gift that cows, chickens, trees, and plants have chosen to share with us? What if we experience our receiving of that food as the acceptance of a gift created by wind and water, flesh and blood, sun and soil? What if we go on to experience our own gratitude for this gift, if that gratitude then becomes a desire to share the gift with others, through the work we do and the love we offer? In this spiritual view, the very process of digestion becomes a transformation, in which the Desire to Receive for the Self Alone becomes a Desire to Receive for the Sake of Sharing.

Based on this perspective, I urged Eleanor to view eating not as a mechanical necessity but, rather, as a part of the flow of life. In this way of thinking, it's no wonder that anything impeding that flow—eating too rapidly, too greedily, or without pleasure in the gift we have received—is bound to cause problems for our digestion and our health.

Interestingly, the Hebrew word *Satan*—the kabbalistic code word for negative forces—comes from the same root as the verb *to impede*. Satan, in this view, is not a devil or a demon, but simply any internal or external force that impedes the flow of energy and love that is otherwise abundantly available to us. We access this flow every time we eat—and so every encounter with food is a profoundly charged occasion. Thus, within the Matrix, eating is never a neutral act. Either we see the divine in food and relate to it accordingly, allowing ourselves to share in the flow of life, or we fall prey to Satan and block the flow. We can continually remind ourselves that food is part of the flow of giving and receiving, the dance of sharing between the natural world and ourselves, between ourselves and each other. Or we can eat out of the desire to receive for ourselves alone, treating animals, plants, and the earth itself with contempt, forgetting that we are all part of the same giant ecosystem, the same perpetual interplay of giving and receiving.

Looked at in this way, eating becomes a form of meditation, in which the magic, the wonder, and eventually the divine aspects of food are allowed to emerge. In this perspective, too, healthy habits of eating become second nature, an obvious way to relate to the gift we are consuming. Chewing each bite of food 40 to 100 times, for example, is a medically accepted way to maximize nutrition and support digestion. Such chewing breaks open the cells, releasing enzymes that are crucial for human digestion. The more enzymes that are released, the more thoroughly we are able to absorb the nutrients we ingest, consuming less food for the same nutritional benefit.

This process of mastication may seem tedious if our focus is on satisfying our hunger—our Desire to Receive for the Self Alone. But if we experience the food as a gift that nature has shared with us, it becomes natural to chew it thoroughly, savoring every bite and focusing on all its benefits. This message was very well understood by the Essenes, a religious community of which Jesus was a member and which created an alternate set of gospels known as the Essene Gospels. In the words of the Essene Jesus, in The Essene Gospel of Peace, Book One:

And when you eat, have above you the angel of air, and below you that angel of water. Breathe long and deeply at all your meals, that the angel of air may bless your repasts. And chew well your food with your teeth, that it becomes water, and that the angel of water turns it into blood in your body. And eat slowly, as if it were a prayer you make to the Lord. For I tell you truly, the power of God enters into you if you eat after this manner at his table. . . .

FREE RADICALS AND INFLAMMATION

Take heed unto thyself and take care of thy life.

—DEUTERONOMY 4:9

At this point, I feel obliged to stress that, despite the spiritual terms in which I'm speaking, I am making these observations *as a physician*. It is my medical opinion, as well as my spiritual belief, that a mechanistic relationship to food is unhealthy not just for our souls but also for our bodies, and that a deeper understanding of nutrition and anatomy will inevitably lead us back to these spiritual themes.

For example, one of the major issues in modern nutrition is the question of free radicals—molecules that become unstable because they are missing one or more electrons. When oxygen becomes unstable in this way, it turns from a healthy, life-giving necessity to a dangerous, possibly life-threatening element. The process that results is known as *oxidation,* which, when we encounter it in metals, we also call "rust." Just as old metal becomes rusty, so does the gradual oxidation of our tissues create the phenomenon of aging.

Although it occurs on a molecular level, the oxidation process is a violent one. An oxygen molecule that is missing an electron will, through electrical force, rip an electron out of a neighboring atom. The neighbor then becomes a free radical itself, engaging in its own "electron raid" as it pulls an electron from yet another atom. The resulting chain reaction leads to a vast increase in the production of free radicals, which can lead in turn to inflammation. And as Randolph learned in Chapter 4, this inflammation is associated with heart disease as well as arthritis, asthma, allergies and other autoimmune disorders, gastrointestinal problems, chronic infection, and cancer. Free radicals are the result as well as the cause of inflammation, helping to create yet another vicious circle in which the results of inflammation further inflame the system.

Is not this image of a molecule tearing out an electron from its neighbor a perfect expression of the kabbalistic principle of Receiving for the Self Alone? And the antidote—the antioxidants to be found in brightly colored fresh fruits, vegetables, and herbs, as well as in fish and in some other food sources—is an equally apt expression of the principle of sharing. The antioxidants don't destroy free radicals but, rather, help supply them with the elements they need to balance their electrical charges, interrupting the process of electron raids and allowing the various elements of the body to work in harmony with one another.

Of course, no scientific studies yet exist to demonstrate the relationship between our attitudes toward food and the production of free radicals. Yet we know that when ulcer patients become angry during their meals, their ulcer symptoms worsen, and we know that eating too fast and not chewing properly can lead to indigestion, acid reflux, and other gastrointestinal problems. Several years as a doctor enable me to say without hesitation, when my patients' attitude toward food shifts, their health improves.

Eleanor was a striking example. As she gradually adopted a friendlier relationship to food, she reported far less difficulty keeping both her weight and her blood sugars at healthy levels. More important, she began to enjoy eating and to see her physical self as a source of pleasure rather than as a constant danger.

FOOD CHOICES IN THE MATRIX

> Everything in the world has a hidden meaning.... Men, ani-
> mals, trees, stars, they are all hieroglyphics.... When you
> see them, you do not understand them. You think they are
> really men, animals, trees, stars. It is only years later...
> that you understand.
>
> —NIKOS KAZANTZAKIS, *ZORBA THE GREEK*

Frequently, patients ask me for meal plans—ready-made dietary choices that they can simply follow blindly, secure in the knowledge that they are practicing good nutrition.

In my previous book, *Gut Reactions,* I offered a number of specific menus to help people with various gastrointestinal disorders learn how to rethink their relationship to food. In this book, however, I'd rather help you learn to enter into the consciousness from which healthy food choices are made. Once you've learned what food signifies and how to eat consciously, you'll be able to tune in to your greater awareness, making the perfect choices for yourself at any given time.

So let's begin with what the novelist Nikos Kazantzakis has called the "hidden meanings" of food—the "hieroglyphics" that nature has given us to read. As we saw in Chapter 3, green is the color of *Tiferet,* the *Sefirot* located around the heart that represents the synthesis of the Desire to Share and the Desire to Receive. Green is, therefore, considered a healing color, and so green foods—such as kale, collards, kohlrabi, chard, beet greens, and mustard greens—are also extremely healthy. One way to improve your energy and boost your immune system is to increase your intake of fresh greens, lightly steamed, perhaps with a little lemon, garlic, or tamari.

Greens are also a rich source of calcium. Many of us need to cut back our consumption of dairy products, especially milk, cheese, and butter. Dairy products tend to be high in fat, and even reduced-fat or nonfat milks and cheeses can trigger food sensitivities, cravings, and problems with digestion.

If you do cut back on dairy products, however, it's important to replenish your calcium intake with several servings of fresh greens each week. A high intake of greens has a cleansing, detoxifying effect on the body, and can create an energized feeling of lightness, as opposed to the bloated, sluggish feeling that often results from a high consumption of dairy products. Eleanor, for example, noticed that when she cut back on her consumption of milk and cheese, and increased her intake of fresh greens, she felt "freer and lighter," as she put it. She told me that she felt mentally freer as well, that she no longer experienced the intense cravings for milk and cheese that had helped her feel like "a slave to food."

Green is not the only color associated with healing. In recent years, we've come to understand that color in food is a clue both to certain nutrients—such as the association of orange foods with beta-carotene—and to flavonoids, plant pigments that support health in a variety of ways. Some flavonoids strengthen capillaries and other connective tissue, while others fight inflammation, histamines (the irritating hormones linked to allergic reactions), and viruses. Recent nutritional research has found that some flavonoids have antioxidant properties, while others have been linked with possible effects against diabetes, cataracts, and even cancer.

From a kabbalistic perspective, every color has a different meaning and a different association with the *Sefirot*. So again, it makes sense that we should seek out food with the most intense coloring, which is likely to be the highest in antioxidants and flavonoids. By the same token, we should avail ourselves of the full range of nutrients by consuming as wide a variety of pigments as possible: red berries, beets, and tomatoes; orange carrots, sweet potatoes, and yams; purple eggplant and grapes; and of course, fresh green peas, broccoli, and leafy greens. Green herbs—including fresh parsley, dill, sage, mint, and coriander— are also high in flavonoids and have many healing properties.

Seeds and nuts are considered extremely powerful in the kabbalistic tradition because they contain in concentrated form the entire blueprint for the grown plant. Thus, seeds provide us with high doses of energy that in Kabbalah are associated with *Keter,* the *Sefir* at the crown of the head. Interestingly, nutritionists find that seeds and nuts are excellent brain food, helping to provide the nutrients we need to support the hormones, neurotransmitters, and biochemicals that sharpen our thoughts and balance our emotions.

Sea vegetables and seaweed are also healing foods. From a kabbalistic perspective, this is not surprising, since water represents *Chesed,* the principle of sharing. Because water is so central to Matrix Healing, I've devoted all of the following chapter to that topic, so let me focus here on plants or animals that live in water, which are naturally healthy means of sharing in nature's bounty. Sea vegetables tend to be even higher in calcium than earthly greens, and they are also a rich source of iodine. Moreover, they possess the power to neutralize toxins, radioactivity, and other environmental insults that can produce free radicals and lead to inflammation.

Fish, which live in water, are also an extremely healthy food. The American Heart Association has recently begun to recommend eating fatty fish at least twice a week, to benefit from their high levels of omega-3 fatty acids. Although for many years, mainstream doctors argued that a high-fat diet was generally unhealthy, and particularly so for people prone to heart disease, conventional medicine is finally beginning to catch up with those pioneering nutritionists who talked about different types of fats, pointing out that the body needs a certain balance between omega-6 fats (found in meat, poultry, and corn, among other sources) and omega-3 fats (found in fish, soy, and flax, among other sources). Fast foods and packaged foods tend to contain extremely high levels of omega-6 fats and hydrogenated fats (hydrogenation is a preservation process that keeps fat from becoming rancid but also makes it an extremely unhealthy substance). So we can benefit from the healing power of the sea by increasing our intake of foods rich in omega-3 fatty acids while cutting fast foods and packaged foods from our diets.

Shellfish, on the other hand, are bottom feeders, living on the waste and garbage that they find on the ocean floor. So it should be no surprise that they are a less healthy food, higher than fish in cholesterol and the wrong types of fat. Shrimp are particularly high in cholesterol and so are generally not recommended for people who are prone to heart disease or vascular problems.

Meat is a more complicated question in the Matrix. In recent years, we've all become more aware of the health problems that can result from excessive consumption of red meat. Ecologists have also drawn our attention to the social problems with meat-eating, pointing out that one acre of land yields only 165 pounds of beef protein—but might produce 20,000 pounds of potatoes. According to Gabriel Cousens, M.D., writing in *Conscious Eating,* more than 80 percent of U.S. corn and 95 percent of U.S. oats are fed to livestock. Meanwhile, people concerned with the treatment of animals have exposed the horrendous conditions in farms and slaughterhouses, pointing out that a violent, painful death is not only cruel to the animal but also unhealthy for the person who eats the resulting meat, which is laden with stress hormones and other toxins released by the animal before its death.

From a kabbalistic perspective, it's impossible not to believe that we will be affected by the way we treat the animals we eat. Today we treat animals as objects, raising them in pens so small they can't move. It has become more important to have tender meat and profitable farms than to allow animals a healthy, natural existence. As a result, corporate farm animals' lives, as well as their deaths, are marked by unnecessary cruelty—a cruelty that I believe must boomerang back upon ourselves, so that on some level we experience their suffering when we eat their flesh. Is it any wonder that excessive meat consumption in the United States is linked to heart disease, hormonal problems, and cancer? That the hormones given to cows and chickens are loading our livers with toxins that inflame our entire systems? That the incidence and number of autoimmune diseases is on the rise? If we believe in the kabbalistic notion of a single universal ecosystem— a single flow of spiritual and physical energy among all of creation—we must see that the cruelty we extend to the animals we eat will inevitably return to haunt our own bodies.

Having said this, I am not opposed to meat-eating per se. Indeed, studies have shown that the healthiest people are those who eat small amounts of meat along with a predominantly vegetarian diet—meat used as one minor element in a sauce or a stew, a few ounces of meat added to a dish of rice and beans or as flavoring for a vegetable dish. However, the meat we eat should be free-range and cruelty-free—or our bodies will pay the price.

THE HIDDEN MESSAGE OF FOOD

Restraint everywhere is excellent.

—BUDDHA

One of the most important kabbalists of the nineteenth century was a rabbi and scholar known as the Ari. Because food is such a central aspect of our participation in the universal flow of energy, the Ari wrote extensively on the nature of food. Much of his writing focused on the notion of "elevating the sparks," flowing from the kabbalists' vision of the universe as brimming over with divine sparks of energy that fell into the physical world during its initial creation. (You can read more about Kabbalah's version of the Big Bang in Chapter 2.) Kabbalists believe that these sparks exist throughout all creation, but because we are not yet ready to see them, they lurk within shells known in Hebrew as *Kleipot*. Our goal is to learn to recognize these sparks, however hidden they may be, and to elevate them—to release them from their shells.

The Ari took this notion of *Kleipot* and applied it to fruits and vegetables. Because the Ari believed that everything in the universe could be understood in terms of its relationship to giving, he classified foods into four categories, so that we could view food not as fuel for our engines but, rather, as a manifestation of the basic universal themes of sharing and receiving:

1. **Fully surrendered:** Strawberries, blueberries, figs, carrots, greens, broccoli, potatoes, beets, seedless grapes. These are the portion of nature's bounty that offers bounty without reservation. They have no skin, peel, pits, or seeds to impede their giving nature. They simply offer themselves unconditionally, manifesting the unconditional sharing that is possible for us if we learn from their example.

2. **Poorly defended:** Dates, plums, olives, apples, peaches, pears, grapes with seeds. These fruits and vegetables have no outer shell but they do protect their inner selves with a pit. They give freely at first, but ultimately, hold back a bit. If the first type of fruit and vegetable represents the ultimate type of spiritual sharing—free-flowing, with no boundaries of any type—this second type of food combines physicality and spirituality. It also manifests the principle of restraint—the restricted giving that is sometimes necessary, as we saw in Chapter 3.

3. **Defended:** Walnuts, coconuts, pineapples, legumes. The foods in this category protect themselves with a tough outer shell whose strength and solidity enables them to let go of the inner protection of the pit. They remind us of the heart, which is totally open at its core yet resides within a tough, protective layer of fat. In this earthly life, sometimes we must defend ourselves. Yet even as we hide our true natures behind a protective coating, we must be ready to reveal them to the people who are wise and loving enough to penetrate our deceptive outer shells and discover the rich, sweet nourishment beneath.

   Defended foods also remind us that restrictions and limitations are sometimes necessary for life to proceed. Yes, it takes a lot of work to strip away the pineapple's outer husk, but without that protective shell, the fruit would be too vulnerable and we would not have the ability to enjoy it.

4. **Highly defended:** Oranges, grapefruits, avocado. These foods contain both inner and outer protection, both a tough outer shell and a pit or pits within. Interestingly, these foods are very dense and rich in nourishment, adding important nutrients to the diet in small amounts. Yet eating too much of them can cause problems. They, too, represent the need for restriction, for temporarily restraining our receiving in order to gain greater benefits in the long run. Just as the

right-column *Sefira* of *Chesed,* or mercy, must be tempered
by the left-column *Sefira* of *Gevurah,* or severe judgment, so
must the open, unconditional sharing of berries and greens
be balanced by the more measured and challenging gifts of
avocados and citrus fruits.

The point of the Ari's analysis was not to privilege certain fruits
and vegetables above others, but rather to help us see Kazantzakis's point: that even the food we eat is as much hieroglyphic as
nourishment—or, rather, it offers nourishment through its sym-
bolic nature as well as through its physical being. An integral part
of Matrix Healing is learning to see these themes throughout our
world, and particularly in the food we eat.

When Eleanor heard the Ari's analysis, she was powerfully
shaken to think that every fruit and vegetable carried such profound messages. She was particularly fond of strawberries, and
she told me that the experience of eating one would never be the
same again.

I told her that in order to better read the message in each bit
of food I eat, I prefer raw foods to cooked ones, and foods served
separately or in large, recognizable chunks to foods that are
blended together. When I recognize each bite I take, I can focus
more fully on each type of food, becoming intimate with its special theme and messages, seeing it as satisfying both my physical
and my spiritual hunger.

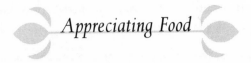

Appreciating Food

PREPARATION

Although you can do this exercise any time you eat—and ideally, will come to do it every time you eat—begin with a meal that you or someone you love has prepared. Create a calm, uninterrupted hour for the meal, and try to use only fresh, organic fruit, vegetables, grains, fish, and/or meat. Try to prepare a meal with a range of colors and textures, and to serve foods that are either raw or have been very lightly cooked. Prepare the meal in such a way that you can spend a few minutes eating only one type of food—say, a tomato and avocado salad, broiled fish, brown rice, and steamed greens. Serve the meal in an attractive way in a peaceful and well-ordered setting.

MEDITATION

1. Focus on the first ingredient—let's say, a tomato. Think about it growing on the vine; see the sun hitting it as the water droplets form early in the morning. Think about the farmer who grew the tomato; envision the labor he or she performed, the energy and effort that went into plowing the dirt, planting the seeds, pulling the weeds. As you eat the tomato, think of yourself as developing a relationship with every element that helped create it—sun, soil, wind, water, human labor. Feel yourself absorbing the gifts of nature and of other humans—gifts that have resulted in your being able to eat this food and absorb its nutrients.

2. Now focus on the tomato itself—its color, its texture, its taste, its scent. As you chew, envision the molecules and atoms in the tomato. Get in touch with the tomato's nutrients and pigment, and experience the nourishment it is sharing with you. Allow yourself to chew each bite from 40 to 100 times. With each grinding of your teeth, see the cells of the tomato breaking open. Feel them

releasing their nutrients. Feel your own body receiving, absorbing, and appreciating this nourishment.

3. Experience your own newly acquired strength and energy. Allow yourself to enjoy the blood streaming through your vessels, the sturdy tissue being built up within your bones, the biochemicals transmitting thoughts and emotions through your brain. Feel your gratitude for the way this food is sharing this strength and energy with you.

4. Continue this meditation with every other ingredient in the meal. When the meal is over, sit quietly for a few minutes and check in with your body and your emotions. How do you feel, physically, mentally, and spiritually, now that you have eaten in this way? How is it different from how you usually feel after a meal? How is it the same? What parts of this eating experience would you like to re-create the next time you eat?

SUGAR: RECEIVING FOR THE SELF ALONE

> Woe unto them that call evil good and good evil; that put darkness for light and light for darkness; that put bitter for sweet and sweet for bitter!
>
> —ISAIAH

One of Eleanor's greatest frustrations as she struggled with her food choices was her intense craving for sugar and sweetened foods. As a diabetic, Eleanor knew that she had to be especially careful about such foods, partly because they contributed to weight gain but even more because they prevented her from maintaining nice, even levels of blood sugar. Instead, high-sugar foods created a pattern of spikes and crashes in her blood-sugar level—the "sugar highs and lows" that are bad for everybody's health, but downright dangerous for people with diabetes.

"I hate knowing that even if I lost a lot of weight, I *still* wouldn't be able to eat all the desserts I wanted," Eleanor told me. "It feels so unfair knowing that this treat will be out of my reach forever, no matter what I do."

I could certainly sympathize. Most of us have felt intense cravings for sweets at some time in our lives, not least because, in this world of packaged foods, some type of sweetener is added to virtually everything that comes in a bottle, box, or jar. Even foods like ketchup, unfrosted cereals, and canned vegetables often contain some form of sugar, corn syrup, or molasses. And this unremitting diet of sugar-sweetened foods can create a constant craving for sugar that can come to feel like an addiction.

Yet I also knew that virtually all of my patients, diabetic or not, would benefit from maintaining balanced blood-sugar levels and cutting back on the sweeteners in their diets. Angelita's migraines (Chapter 3), Randolph's heart condition (Chapter 4), even the cancer of patients like Joan (Chapter 1) and Mitchell (Chapter 2), have all been associated with a high intake of processed sugar and the consequent spikes and crashes in blood-sugar levels. Even my patients who are technically healthy experience debilitating effects from eating too much sugar: fatigue, irritability, memory problems, foggy thinking, mood swings, menstrual problems, weight gain and weight retention, and an overall loss in energy and well-being.

Let's take a closer look at the biology of sugar. Everything we eat is translated by our digestive systems into glucose, or blood sugar, which travels throughout our bloodstreams, energizing every cell in our bodies. If we take in more nutrients than we need at any one time, the excess glucose is converted to glycogen and stored in our livers. There, it is available for when we get hungry, to hold us over until the next meal.

The glucose in our bloodstream can't be used, however, until it is further metabolized by the hormone insulin, which is produced in the pancreas. A rise in blood-sugar levels triggers a release of insulin, which metabolizes the glucose, causing our blood-sugar levels to fall. When our blood-sugar levels fall low enough, we start to feel hungry, prompting us to eat again. The new meal causes our blood-sugar levels to rise—and the whole process starts all over again.

This system works best when we are continually but gradually replenishing our glucose stores with natural foods. Meat, fish, fruit, vegetables, and unprocessed grains (that is, grains that have not yet been turned into flour) all metabolize into glucose relatively slowly. This is why eating four to six small meals is a healthier choice than three large meals—and why eating regularly is far better than skipping a meal. Our bodies function at their highest levels when they are continually supplied—but not oversupplied—with the glucose that they need.

What happens if our glucose levels drop and we *don't* eat? To keep us from starving to death, our livers convert their glycogen into glucose to keep our blood sugar at an acceptable level until we eat again. You can see why it's better, though, never to get too hungry, and never to get too full. Rather than asking your liver to convert excess blood sugar into glycogen, and then to convert the glycogen back into glucose, it's better simply to stock your blood with glucose through small, regular, nutritious meals.

When I say not to get too hungry, I'm not referring to the pleasant sensation of being eager to eat. I'm talking about the kind of uncomfortable hunger that goes with genuinely low blood sugar (hypoglycemia), which can create such symptoms as shakiness, dizziness, nervousness, sweating, irritability, and heart pounding. Some people feel forgetful, foggy, and vague when their blood sugar falls too low. Others begin to develop headaches.

These symptoms disappear as soon as you take in more food. But what happens when the food you ingest is high in processed sugar or refined carbohydrates—a candy bar, pastry, or even a piece of whole wheat bread?

Sugars and refined carbohydrates are very quickly converted into glucose—far more quickly than the nutrients in meat, fish, fruits, vegetables, and unprocessed grains. So when you eat a sweet snack, or one made from refined flour, your blood sugar spikes quickly and triggers a larger-than-normal surge in insulin. This excess insulin metabolizes your blood sugar very quickly, and suddenly your blood sugars have fallen too far, too fast. In other words, when you eat sugar, first you get the sugar rush that comes from a spike in your blood sugars. Then you get the crash that comes from excess insulin metabolizing your blood sugar too quickly.

Although diabetes is to some extent an inherited disease, it can also be triggered, worsened, or even engendered by this cycle of high blood sugar and hyperproduction of insulin. Exhausted from making too much insulin, the pancreas begins to have trouble making it at all, which can eventually lead to glucose intolerance (difficulty metabolizing glucose) and then to full-out diabetes.

Even those of us not at risk for diabetes itself suffer from this process, however. Spiking and falling blood-sugar levels put a strain on the liver, as that organ attempts to maintain normal glucose/glycogen levels. The process is also a major migraine trigger. It contributes to the inverse of diabetes, a condition known as hypoglycemia, in which even the slightest sensation of hunger triggers extreme symptoms of irritability, anxiety, or confusion. The excess production of insulin contributes to weight gain and weight retention, even among people who diet strenuously and exercise regularly. And the endless round of highs and crashes prevents us from enjoying a balanced sense of energy and well-being.

As a diabetic, Eleanor was familiar with most of the biological aspects of the blood-sugar cycle. What she didn't know, however, was that the kabbalists view consuming sugar as the ultimate expression of the Desire to Receive for the Self Alone. Eating more nutritious foods represents the synthesis of receiving and sharing—the Desire to Receive for the Sake of Sharing. The empty calories of sugar, however, do not trigger the same expansive sense of well-being, the balanced energy that seeks to share through love and work. Rather, sugar engenders only greed for more sugar, an endless Desire to Receive for the Self Alone that can never really be satisfied.

From this point of view, I think it is no accident that sugar developed in conjunction with the international slave trade and the New World system of slavery. The mass production of sugar was only made possible because of the sugarcane plantations in the Caribbean, in which European colonists used forced African labor to grow the immensely profitable new crop. The slavery on the sugar islands was some of the cruelest that has ever existed, based on a system in which slaves were "used up" quickly and then replaced with new purchases from Africa. For most of Caribbean history, Africans brought to the islands survived an average of only three years.

Life for the colonists was not much healthier. The rich European owners of the sugarcane plantations considered work and exercise to be the province of their slaves, while their own idleness was seen as a badge of honor. Moreover, they insisted on maintaining European styles of dress and architecture, which were completely unsuitable for the tropical climate. They had no resistance to the diseases of the islands or to those that the enslaved Africans brought with them. And the colonists were notorious for eating large, heavy meals and drinking huge quantities of rum and other alcoholic beverages—all high in sugar, all conspicuous displays of wealth and status that were also extremely bad for their health.

Although relatively little sugarcane was grown in North America (except for in the French colony Louisiana), much of North America's economy relied upon slavery. Colonists in what would eventually become the U.S. South bought enslaved Africans in the international market created to supply the Caribbean colonies. Northern colonies, especially New England and New York, depended on trade with the slave islands. Because sugarcane was such a valuable crop, Caribbean colonists preferred to buy their foodstuffs and basic goods from North America, rather than diverting land or labor from the profitable cultivation of sugarcane.

Once we know that sugar represents the Desire to Receive for the Self Alone, we have no trouble understanding why sugarcane cultivation became a veritable engine of greed in the New World, gobbling up land that might otherwise have been used to grow healthy food; inspiring traders and growers to treat human beings like objects; creating a culture based on conspicuous consumption and unhealthy habits. No wonder that sugar inspires cravings that cannot be satisfied, that it causes multiple problems for our health and our weight, that it impedes the flow of life-giving energy within our bodies. Yes, of course it tastes good! But if we practice what Gabriel Cousens calls "conscious eating," remaining aware of what we eat and how it affects us, our craving for sugar can begin to dull.

That at least was Eleanor's experience. Knowing how sugar affected her body was only partly helpful. What really made the difference, she told me, was realizing what sugar meant in the larger scheme of things—how it had affected the balance of the world's energy and what kind of energy it brought into her own body. "I hate to say it," she remarked at a recent appointment, "but those sweet desserts really just don't taste as good to me anymore. I'm not saying I never eat them. But they certainly don't have the same hold on me that they used to."

ALCOHOL, CAFFEINE, AND OTHER STIMULANTS: CRAVING THE BREAD OF SHAME

> Think of the wonders uncorked by wine! It opens secrets, gives heart to our hopes, pushes the cowardly into battle, lifts the load from anxious minds, and evokes talents. Thanks to the bottle's prompting no one is lost for words, no one who's cramped by poverty fails to find release.
>
> —HORACE

Eleanor was well aware that alcohol, caffeine, nicotine, and recreational drugs can overstress and toxify the liver, as can many over-the-counter and prescription medications. As we saw in Chapter 4, a toxic liver can intensify allergies and autoimmune conditions, and perhaps promote the growth of cancer. And when the liver isn't working at peak efficiency, it doesn't effectively metabolize the fat in our bloodstream, leading to high blood pressure, clogged arteries, heart disease—and weight gain.

By the time she came to me, Eleanor already had a good understanding of this basic biology. What she didn't have was a kabbalistic perspective, in which the liver is seen as the seat of reactive behavior, including anger, frustration, envy, and despair. It was a revelation to Eleanor that there were links between her liver, her diet, and the negative emotions with which she struggled daily, including resentment concerning her diabetes, her food choices, and her weight.

Eleanor was also fascinated to discover that kabbalists see alcohol, caffeine, and even some medications as aspects of the Bread of Shame. As we saw in Chapter 2, the Bread of Shame is what caused the first Vessel to push back against the Light, refusing the Light's bountiful sharing. While the Vessel wanted to receive the good things that the Light had to offer, it was also ashamed of not being able to give in return. Indeed, the entire material universe was created so that the Vessel could eventually move beyond the Bread of Shame, becoming fully giving and wholly empowered—becoming, in fact, exactly like the Light.

Artificial stimulants and medications make us feel good in the short run, but they, too, evoke the Bread of Shame. Although, as Horace points out, they enable us to accomplish goals that are otherwise outside our reach and are sometimes even crucial to our health, they carry with them the shame that we are not able to achieve these goals on our own. While caffeine, alcohol, and certain medications may be fine in moderation, it's useful to remember that we pay a price for their good effects—a price that represents our deepest wish to achieve our goals entirely through our own efforts.

As Eleanor learned more about the hidden meanings of food, she began to discover that shifting her diet could also affect her mood, her behavior, and her sense of herself. She already understood the health reasons for detoxifying her liver, and she was pleased to discover that supporting her liver would make it easier to control her weight. But she was even more excited by the prospect of creating a more peaceful and satisfying life, one that was not so marked with envy, anger, and frustration. For Eleanor, shifting both her diet and her relationship to food evoked my favorite passage from the Zohar: "Open to me an opening no bigger than the eye of a needle, and I will open to you the heavenly gates."

HUNGER AND CHARITY

> A group of people were sitting in a lifeboat, when they were surprised by one of the passengers. He calmly took out a drill and began drilling a hole in the floor of the boat.
>
> "Are you crazy? We'll sink! Stop that this instant!" the other passengers cried—but the man shook his head and kept drilling.
>
> "It's really none of your business," he said coolly. "After all, I'm only drilling under my own seat."
>
> —JEWISH FOLKTALE

Whenever I speak with my patients about food and diet, I'm struck by a powerful paradox. On the one hand, each of us is responsible for his or her own health—based on the food we eat, the emotions we feel, the actions we take. On the other hand, we are all part of something larger—a body and soul that we share with all of creation. Although it would seem that each of us has perfect health within our grasp, ultimately, none of us is healed until we all are.

Nowhere does this paradox strike me more powerfully than with issues of food and hunger. Can it be an accident that while millions of people are starving throughout the world, we in the United States are literally dying from our own abundance—from the excess calories, fat, sugar, and salt that we consume each day, from the pollutants and toxins released into the environment in our pursuit of luxury and wealth?

The number-one health problem in the world today is not AIDS or cancer or some other incurable disease. It's chronic malnutrition, a problem that could be solved merely by the redistribution of the earth's abundant food. Yet according to the United Nations, half of the world's population suffers from some form of malnutrition, with 800 million people seriously malnourished. At least 25 percent of the world's children suffer from lack of food, and 42,000 children die each day because they don't have enough to eat. In fact, malnourished children account for 15 million deaths each year—or 30 percent of all the world's yearly deaths. In the last ten years, more people have died from malnutrition than from all the wars and murders of the last 150 years.

So I would finally say to anyone who is concerned about his or her own diet, weight, and relationship to food: feed the hungry and your own health will benefit. Again, that's not a religious or even a spiritual statement as much as a medical one. If you truly give of yourself to try to end the problem of world hunger, I guarantee that your own relationship to food will improve. Otherwise, ultimately, all our efforts to improve our diets and our nutrition come to resemble the activity of the man in the folktale. In this world, there's no such thing as drilling just under our own seat. We're all in the lifeboat together.

GETTING READY TO EAT

Traditional Judaism requires the devout man to follow a strict routine: he gets up, washes, puts on the prayer shawl, and prays. Then he has breakfast.

But when Paul's son came back from the university, he suddenly refused to follow this pious routine. "Every day I

ask him, and each day he refuses," Paul told his friend Jacob.
"It's been five days now that he refuses to pray."

　　Jacob was horrified. "But if he's not careful, he'll starve,"
he exclaimed. "For God's sake, how long can he hold out?"

　　　　　　　　—TRADITIONAL FOLKTALE ADAPTED FROM *A TREASURY*
　　　　　　　　OF JEWISH FOLKLORE, EDITED BY NATHAN AUSUBEL

Virtually every religion features some form of prayer before eating, and I don't think this is an accident. When I was growing up, I was taught that God needed our acknowledgment at every point in the day, including at mealtimes. Now I understand that the Creator couldn't care less whether we acknowledge Him or Her. Rather, *we* are impoverished if we forget that eating creates a larger relationship between us and the rest of the universe, if we allow our hunger to override our greater sense of sharing. To quote from Gabriel Cousens, M.D., once again:

> *To experience oneself as interwoven with nature leads to receiving our food with more love and gratefulness. If food is eaten with a prayer of gratitude and respect for the life force it bestows and the sacrifice it is making for the survival of the human body, the food will carry the love of this prayer inside. The power and sacredness of the eating process are enhanced by the awareness that each particular fruit or vegetable is giving up its own individual existence as part of the evolutionary process so that it may be assimilated into the greater existence of the human body. In this larger context, eating becomes a sacred act. . . .*

My mentor, Rabbi Berg, puts it another way: "The most important part of eating is the initial restriction." Restriction in this sense is not the punitive calorie-counting of so many fad diets, nor is it an ascetic unwillingness to enjoy the tastes, smells, and textures of food. Rather, it is a moment of prayer and reflection taken before eating, to help transmute our Desire to Receive for the Self Alone into a Desire to Receive for the Sake of Sharing.

To this end, I believe that every act of eating should begin with a moment of meditation. You don't have to follow the routine of pious Jews and put on a prayer shawl, nor do you have to say the words of a traditional grace. But if you restrict your initial hunger by taking the time to remember why you are eating and how you are a being larger than your physical appetites, you will find that your health, digestion, and relationship to food improve. You may even find that you enjoy your mealtimes more!

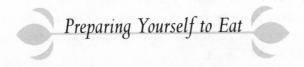

Preparing Yourself to Eat

PREPARATION

While you ideally will learn to do some version of this meditation every time you eat, you might find it easiest to begin practicing this approach at a meal prepared by you or someone you love, eaten in your home or some other space where you feel comfortable. Allow yourself a calm, uninterrupted hour for your meal, and serve the food in an attractive way in a peaceful and well-ordered setting. As you become proficient in this type of before-meal meditation, you can find ways to adapt it to different settings and circumstances.

MEDITATION

1. Focus on the energy and resources that had to be mobilized to bring this food to your table. See the labor of the farmworkers, the truckers, the workers in the grocery store. Silently thank the people involved in bringing this food to you, and promise them that you will make good use of their energy and care.

2. Visualize the natural processes that created the food on your table—the sun and soil, the wind and water, the strength of the plants growing upward, despite the downward pull of gravity. Get in touch with the energy of the sap carrying nutrients up from the soil to every part of the plant, with the creativity and generosity of the plant that produces root, stem, leaves, flowers, fruit, and seeds. See each item of food in its natural habitat, and feel the energy pulsing throughout the natural world that brought life to your food and now is bringing life to you.

3. Experience your own body, its hunger and its strength, its energy and its desires. Feel your own blood coursing through your veins, the continual replenishment of your bones, the dance of biochemicals that transmit your thoughts, emotions, and desires. If you have a particular area of concern in your health, visualize the part of your body or the anatomical system that needs special nurturing and support.

4. Imagine, just before you eat, the relief and gratitude and joy with which your body will greet the nourishment you are about to provide. Promise yourself and the world that created this food that you will make good use of this nourishment, that you will consecrate this human and natural energy to a great purpose— allowing you to enjoy your life, sharing your love with family and friends, expressing your inner truth, working for a better world.

5. Begin to eat. As you take each bite, try to sense the energy of the food and your own energy. Experience the gift you are receiving and your own commitment to making good use of that gift.

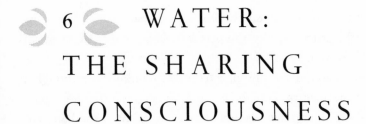

6 WATER: THE SHARING CONSCIOUSNESS

I will bless your bread and water and remove sickness from your midst.

WHEN Teresa burst into my office for the first time, I was struck by what an enthusiastic person she was. A large woman dressed in vivid colors, she seemed to fill the room with her eager questions, her attentive gaze, and her warm, hearty laugh. She paused to chat with the nurses at the front desk, who happened to be having an unusually busy and stressful day—and within a few minutes, the whole mood in the office had lightened. As I was saying good-bye to my previous patient, I noticed that Teresa had struck up a conversation with an elderly man sitting beside her in the waiting area, and soon he, too, was laughing and talking animatedly to her. The term *generosity of spirit* seemed made to order for this exuberant, lively woman.

Yet as I came to know her, I found there was another side to Teresa, a small and anxious side that was constantly afraid of never having enough. This fear of scarcity seemed to be the dark side to Teresa's buoyancy and generosity, a doubleness that made sense to me when I learned that for the past ten years, Teresa had been suffering from bulimia.

Teresa considered herself a "controlled bulimic." Although in her teenage years, she'd been caught in a constant cycle of binging and purging, she was now in her late twenties and had managed to restrict bulimic episodes to times in her life that were particularly stressful. While Teresa was relieved to have made progress, she was still looking for a way to master her eating disorder, once and for all.

Since Teresa seemed to be such a sharing person, I thought she'd connect to the kabbalistic idea of water as embodying the ultimate "sharing consciousness." Water has always been a significant part of Jewish ritual. There are commandments regulating the washing of the hands—done with the appropriate prayer—before every meal, as well as instructions for women's ritual baths. Jewish fasting requires doing without water, so that breaking one's fast then becomes a joyful reunion with the life-giving properties of both drinking and eating.

Kabbalah accepts these traditional views of water, but it goes one step further in seeing water as the embodiment of the Creator's overwhelming wish to *give*—to literally shower us with love and blessings. Kabbalah views water as the very essence of sharing, flowing where it is needed, soothing and cleansing the body, mind, and spirit.

In my view, Teresa felt anxious both about not getting enough and about getting "too much." I thought focusing on water would help her find balance, so that she could both trust in the Creator's abundance and accept her own right to be filled. I shared with Teresa several rituals involving water and suggested that she use each contact with water as a way to tap into the sharing, loving presence of the Creator, who was longing to fill her with love and light—if only she would allow herself to be filled. I also encouraged her to drink more water, particularly after each meal. The healthy physical properties of water are well known. But I believed that Teresa could also benefit from the spiritual qualities of water, allowing herself to feel "in the flow" of giving and receiving.

Eating disorders are particularly difficult to treat, especially when they've persisted as long as Teresa's had. But over time, Teresa began to find a sense of calm around food. Now when she encountered the stressful moments that formerly would have triggered a cycle of binging and purging, she could use the hand-washing ritual to "wash her anxieties away." Likewise, praying over water and then drinking it reminded her that there would always be "enough" and she would always be entitled to it. I thought that since Teresa was already such a loving, sharing person, perhaps water's greatest gift had been to reveal her own true nature.

THE SACRED ELEMENT

> Where a spring rises or a water flows, there ought we to build altars and offer sacrifices.
>
> —SENECA

As the quote from the Roman poet Seneca suggests, water has been considered a sacred element throughout the ages. Moreover, many cultures have seen water as central to healing. According to Charles Ryrie, in *The Healing Power of Water*, African healers saved water in quartz crystal—a practice that modern scientists now believe made use of the silica in quartz to preserve the water's purity. Likewise, the Chinese, who considered water key to our physical, emotional, mental, and spiritual energies, saved glacial water in jade vases, while the Incas and Aztecs stored their water in obsidian jars.

Sometimes water was revered in the form of sacred rivers, such as the Ganges, or the many sacred springs and wells of Ireland, which villagers would surround with ribbons, trinkets, and other small gifts to acknowledge the local water spirits. This sense of sacredness was often bound up in the understanding that human life—indeed, all life on this planet—began in water. Thus, the Sumerian word *mar* means both "sea" and "womb," and the Sumerian *a* means "water," "sperm," "conception," and "generation." Hindu texts also explain that "Everything was water" as creation began, while in Tantric manuscripts and Ayurvedic healing, water is seen as *prana,* the "breath of life." The Greeks advocated bathing as a general health practice, while the Hebrew letter *Mem* means "mother," "life," "womb," or "sea" and, as we'll see in Chapter 8, is part of the three-letter name of God written as *Mem Hay Shin,* a healing sequence of Hebrew letters.

Water is also traditionally part of many religious rites, including baptism, the purification of sacred places, and the preparation of corpses for burial. Bathing in the water of Lourdes, France, is considered a source of healing miracles by the 6 million people who visit the holy site each year. The Islamic holy city of Mecca is the site of a sacred spring that is an important stop on the Haj pilgrimage that every religious Muslim is supposed to make. During the Jewish holiday of Yom Kippur, the day of atoning for sins, many Jewish communities have adopted the practice of symbolically throwing their sins into the nearest body of water, where they are purified and dissolved, leaving the repentant sinners free to start the new year with a clean slate.

When we look at the scientific understanding of water, we can see why it figures so centrally in world cultures. Some 70 percent of our planet is covered in water, and our adult bodies are 75 percent water. We're even closer to the watery element at birth: newborn bodies are 97 percent water. Even our bones are 22 percent water.

Since both we and the earth are made of water, it makes sense that water would be an important element in our health and healing. It also makes sense that when we pollute the waters of our planet, toxify the water we drink, and deprive our bodies of the hydration they need, our health will suffer. As a physician, it is my sense that improper hydration is a factor in such diseases as asthma, arthritis, skin problems, weight gain, osteoporosis, diabetes, heart disease, and cancer. Drinking more pure water can help patients reduce inflammation, boost the healing power of antioxidants, and help balance our production of hormones and neurotransmitters, the chemical messengers that transmit mental and emotional impulses.

Water connects our planet to the sun and moon, whose strong gravitational forces balance with our own planet's gravity to create the tides. Although the ocean tides are the most dramatic and the easiest to see, the tides affect water everywhere on earth— even a few ounces of water in a teacup or the fluids within our bodies. Through water, our bodies partake of the rhythms of the heavens, as well as being linked to the oceans, seas, and rivers of the earth. They are the perfect expression of the kabbalistic principle of wholeness, in which microcosm and macrocosm echo each other in perpetual harmony.

THE GENEROSITY OF WATER

When Adam and Eve were thrown out of the Garden of Eden, God saw that they truly repented and He took pity on them. "My children," He said, "you are now about to become part of a world full of sorrow and hardship. Although I cannot prevent your suffering, I can give you a gift that will ease your pain. Here is a priceless pearl—a tear. When you are feeling sad or troubled, the tears can fall from your eyes and your hearts will grow lighter."

When Adam and Eve heard these words, they both began to cry, and their tears were the first water that nourished the earth. And so whenever grief overtakes us, we have God's gift of tears to ease our burden.

—ADAPTED FROM THE MIDRASH, THE COMMENTARY ON THE
TALMUD, AND FROM *A TREASURY OF JEWISH FOLKLORE*,
EDITED BY NATHAN AUSUBEL

In the kabbalistic view, the story of Adam and Eve is a code for how we once left Tree of Life consciousness to live in the world of the Tree of Knowledge. The Tree of Knowledge consciousness limits us to a worldview in which we rely on the evidence of our senses, dependent upon our limited perception of here and now, and on the mistaken belief that we are discrete entities who can be understood separately from our planet as a whole. Tree of Life consciousness—which, symbolically, we left behind in Eden and must learn how to regain—is the worldview of the Matrix, of quantum physics, of understanding that our bodies, with their fluids and tides, are only a microcosm of the planet we inhabit.

It is fitting, in this story, that water should be the link between the Creator, human beings, the earth, and the emotion of grief. Whenever we feel organic grief, we lose our ego boundaries and flow—like water—into a state of empathy and compassion, experiencing both our own sorrows and those of all humanity. We cry tears of joy as well, indicating that any profound emotion has the ability to connect us with our most authentic selves, as well as with the Creator, our fellow humans, and our planet.

It is also fitting that tears are portrayed as God's gift to humanity, enabling us to bear our suffering and care for our planet at the same time. Think of the generosity of water and all that it enables. We take life from the waters of the womb; we express our emotions through the medium of tears; we rely on water to nourish our cells, our fields, and our forests. Tiny droplets of water in our lungs enable us to breathe. Water flows into the smallest crevice, molding its shape to whatever surrounds it. Water is the medium in which many other substances dissolve, and yet water generously yields to those other substances, allowing them to determine the flavor, color, and texture of the new liquid.

In kabbalistic tradition, water represents *Chesed,* the principle of giving and sharing. Thus, the Torah—the first five books of the Bible and the foundation of Judaism—are spoken of as water. As Rabbi Chanimah wrote, "Why are the words of the Torah compared to water? For it is written that everyone who thirsts comes for water."

As you read in Chapter 4, Kabbalah considers that the passions of the heart burn so hot that without the cooling breath of the lungs, the flames of the heart would devour not only itself but also the entire world. Part of that cooling mercy comes from the tiny droplets of water in each breath.

Next time you drink a glass of water, or bathe, or shower, or wash your hands, next time you pass a river or a stream, a lake, or an ocean, think of the healing, merciful powers of water. Here's an exercise to help you connect the water in your own body to the generous waters of the planet.

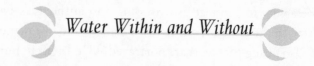

Water Within and Without

PREPARATION

1. Ideally, you will conduct this meditation while sitting beside a body of water—ocean, lake, river, stream, or pool. Whether or not this is possible, fill a glass with water and place it somewhere you can easily see it when you open your eyes.

2. Find a comfortable sitting position, keeping your arms and legs uncrossed so that your right and left sides remain separate. Close your eyes and breathe deeply and slowly. Try to breathe in on a count of eight and out on a count of six, breathing through your nose.

MEDITATION

1. As you breathe, bring your attention deep into your lungs. Become aware of the moisture that you inhale and exhale. Experience the sense of water entering and leaving your body with every breath.

2. Allow your attention to extend to all the water within your body— the fluids in your bloodstream, the tears in your eyes, the liquid in your brain. As you continue to breathe, become aware of the 75 percent of your body that is water.

3. If you are sitting by a body of water, open your eyes. Otherwise, keep your eyes closed and visualize your favorite body of water— an ocean or a river, a stream or a spring. Allow the water you envision to penetrate every one of your senses. See the light play over the water's sparkling surface. Hear the sound it makes lapping against the shore. Smell the salty air or the forest soil. Taste the sweet, fresh water against your tongue or feel the sharp tang of the salt. Feel the cool ocean waves or the icy cold mountain stream. Immerse your senses in the delight of the water.

4. Reconnect to the water within your body as you hold in your senses the experience of water outside your body. Feel yourself as permeable, the same water within and without.

5. Expand your visualization to an image of the entire earth—our planet, Gaia. See the oceans and seas that cover our world, and envision the sun and moon pulling the tides into their ebb and flow.

6. Now, see if you can feel the magnetism of the tides pulling on the waters within your own body. Experience the identity between the water inside your body and the water outside it.

7. Open your eyes and see the nearby glass of water. Continue to hold in your consciousness the sense of the world's water, even as you reach for your own glass of water and slowly drink it. Savor the water you are taking in, even as you feel the pull of the ocean's tides and continue to immerse yourself in the sensory experience of water.

THE MOLECULAR PROPERTIES OF WATER

If there is magic on this planet, it is contained in water.

—LOREN EISLEY, *THE IMMENSE JOURNEY*

You're probably already aware of the fact that water is H_2O: two hydrogen molecules and a single oxygen molecule. But have you ever thought about the amazing fact that these two gases, one of which is lighter than air itself, together form an entirely new substance—the liquid water?

When Teresa and I talked about the nature of water, it was this transformative aspect that meant the most to her. She was especially moved by the notion that hydrogen and oxygen needed to join with one another in order to bring out properties in each element that would never have been apparent had they remained separate. This merging of hydrogen and oxygen into a new element is an excellent example of the physics notion of emergent properties, in which the whole is literally greater than the sum of its parts. Water is not merely the sum of the existing properties of the two gases of which it is composed; rather, the combination of the two elements creates an entirely new set of properties. You might say that hydrogen and oxygen simply "don't know who they are" until they meet each other. And just as we can't truly understand hydrogen and oxygen without knowing about their capacity to form water, we can't understand any human being outside the context of his or her relationships.

"What I like," Teresa told me, "is the idea that these properties were there in hydrogen and oxygen all along, but something new had to come along to bring them out." She blushed and looked down at the floor. "It gives me hope that there are all these new possibilities lurking inside *me*. I just need to figure out how to access them."

From a Matrix Healing point of view, the combination of hydrogen and oxygen indicates a profound truth about our world: that it is only through connection—to other humans, to nature, to the planet itself—that we come into our true natures. As the kabbalists see it, even the Creator had to be in relationship to express His or Her essential nature as a giving, sharing force.

Teresa also enjoyed learning about the vastly different properties of hydrogen and oxygen. Hydrogen, the smallest atom there is, consists of a single positively charged proton at its center, surrounded by a single negatively charged electron rotating around it in three dimensions. The atom is light and unstable. Oxygen is a heavier atom, with eight protons in its center, surrounded by an inner and an outer shell. The inner shell is full—with two electrons orbiting the center. The outer shell has six electrons, but in order to balance the atom's electrical charges, it would "prefer" to contain eight.

The oxygen atom's longing for two extra electrons and the hydrogen atom's essential instability are what enables the marriage of these two substances and the creation of a new element. As Charles Ryrie puts it:

> *Hydrogen can be viewed as a tiny light ethereal body which is very sociable but has a tendency to pull upwards, to aim for the skies. Oxygen is equally sociable but tends to head downwards towards the Earth. At their meeting point they form the universal mediating element, water, with 2 light hydrogen atoms bonding to the heavier oxygen. Water is, if you like, the meeting point between heaven and Earth—it forms a cosmic connection.*

Because hydrogen is so small and light, it can move into the oxygen atom's outer shell more fully than a heavier, more substantial atom might be able to do. In Ryrie's words, "The attraction between them is unusually strong."

Paradoxically, the super-stable element of water is nevertheless able to bond easily with other molecules because of the exchange of electrical charges between the two types of atoms. The oxygen atom pulls the electrons into itself, giving it a slightly negative charge, while the hydrogen atom, having lost its electrons, carries a slightly positive charge. As a result, the hydrogen portion of the water molecule tends to bond with negatively charged atoms and molecules, while the oxygen portion bonds with substances that are positively charged. This bonding property of water enables it to mix with many other substances, which in turn has created many of the conditions for life on earth. It's also a wonderful metaphor for relationships: stable in and of itself, water is nevertheless always ready to mix with another substance and create something new.

The other result of these electrochemical bonds is that water occurs most often as a liquid, rather than a solid substance. If the bonds between the hydrogen and oxygen atoms were only slightly stronger, water would turn solid at 100 degrees Celsius (212 degrees Fahrenheit)—the temperature that is currently its boiling point. Water that froze so easily would make life on earth impossible at anything like its present form.

Let's look a bit more closely at these thermal properties of water. Like all liquids, water starts to shrink as it cools, and logically, you would expect it to continue to shrink, so that ice—the solid form of water—would be denser than its liquid form. Certainly all other liquids behave that way, so that their frozen forms are smaller and more compact than their liquid states.

But water is unique among all the liquids on earth. Although it does shrink until it reaches 4 degrees Celsius (39 degrees Fahrenheit), after that, it begins to expand, so that when water finally freezes at 0 degrees Celsius (32 degrees Fahrenheit), it has created a loosely structured set of molecules—ice that actually takes up *more* space than liquid water, not less.

This odd property of water is a function of the shapes that water molecules take at different temperatures. As a result, an enormous amount of energy is required to freeze water, as well as to boil it. Water seems to resist changing its temperature, and it has a much higher boiling point than virtually all other natural liquids. And when water is at 37 degrees Celsius (99 degrees Fahrenheit), it seems to require the greatest amount of energy to produce a temperature change.

Again, this is lucky for life on earth, specifically for human life. Given that our blood is composed of 90 percent water, this bodily fluid is able to maintain its own steady normal temperature of

98.6 degrees Fahrenheit even when we are subjected to prolonged extremes of heat and cold. Given that our land masses are surrounded by water, our entire planet is insulated from extreme and sudden fluctuations in temperature by the thermal resistance of the ocean, which tends to store and distribute huge amounts of heat, so that the equator's warm temperatures are in a sense shared with northern climes. Charles Ryrie points out that a 100-mile-wide ocean current can transport as much heat in an hour as produced by burning 200 million tonnes of coal.

No wonder the kabbalists consider water to embody the very spirit of sharing! Water transports the vital heat of life throughout our entire planet and helps our bodies—and those of all other living creatures—to maintain their equilibrium. Water helps support life both within our bodies and outside them, sharing its cooling and warming properties wherever they are needed, just as it flows freely into every welcoming crevice and plain.

Teresa told me that she found it enormously calming to meditate on the generosity of water, its seemingly endless ability to provide humans, animals, plants, and the planet itself with whatever they needed. "When I start to feel hungry, or anxious, or inadequate, I breathe deeply, connect to the flow of my own blood, and then bring that awareness outward, so that I feel nurtured and supported by all the seven seas," she said poetically, and then laughed. "I know it sounds extreme, but it's very comforting to think that the entire planet is available to warm me, cool me, and keep my cells floating in a pool of nourishment."

THE HEALING VIBRATIONS OF WATER

> The sage rules with compassion and his word needs to be trusted. The sage needs to know how to flow around blocks, and how to know a way round like water and how to find the way through like water. . . . Water never fights; it flows around without harm.
>
> —TAO TE CHING

One of the most remarkable properties of water is its ability to pick up, retain, and transmit the vibrations of substances with which it comes in contact. Thus, water kept in a plastic container will eventually taste different from water kept in glass or metal. Water can also pick up vibrations from other substances even when it is not in direct contact with them.

If you'd like to see for yourself how this works, put a sealed plastic or glass bottle in your refrigerator next to a ripe melon. After 24 hours, give a glass of this water to your friend and see if he or she can detect an unusual taste. In many cases, the melon flavor will have vibrated its way through the glass or plastic into the water.

As a result of its unusual sensitivity, water picks up information of all types. According to Charles Ryrie, "Water is affected by the chemical information contained in a person's hands, for example—what elements or traces of elements may physically be present on the skin—but also by the very pulse of that person, their rhythmic patterns and vibrations, and vibrations that it picks up from the cosmos, from the Moon and from the planets."

People can also consciously affect the vibrations of water. Canadian researcher Bernard Grad, working in the 1960s, discovered that when a psychic healer held a quantity of water, the seeds irrigated by that water grew more quickly than their neighbors. Likewise, when a depressed person held the same type of water, the seeds it nourished grew more slowly. Grad went on to analyze the properties of the water that the healer had held, and he was able to chart a significant shift in the angle of the hydrogen bond.

You can repeat your own version of Grad's experiment, if you like, following the work of researcher Joseph Bender: pour distilled water into five identical clean glasses and set them out on a table. Choose one glass to hold in your hands as you project loving, healing thoughts into the water for several minutes. Then ask a sample group to taste the water. When Bender conducted several versions of this experiment in Texas, he consistently found that six out of ten adults and nine out of ten children could identify the "loving" water.

Although there is not yet any conventional scientific basis for explaining why this experiment works, Matrix Healing has an explanation. As we saw in Chapter 1, we live in a world of quantum physics, in which human thought can affect the world around us, in which mind can transform matter. Water is an unusually sensitive form of matter that is easily transformed—another indication of its sharing nature.

Teresa was thrilled to find out that she could "sweeten" the water she drank simply by sharing her loving thoughts with it. It seemed clear to both of us that water that had been treated in this way would help magnify the loving, compassionate nature of anyone who drank it, helping us reconnect to our own Desire to Share, to relate freely, and to let our emotions flow. When I taught Teresa the following exercise, she went on to practice it regularly.

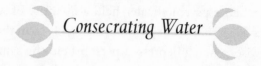

Consecrating Water

PREPARATION

1. Pour the water you wish to "sweeten" into a bottle, pitcher, or glass. (Because of the absorptive power of water, it's best to store it in glass, pottery, or china rather than in plastic or metal.) You can treat a large quantity of water and then refrigerate it, or you can do this exercise glass by glass. It also works with restaurant water or water you receive at another person's house.

2. Take a moment to clear your mind, using a few deep, conscious breaths to clear your thoughts. Tap into your own sense of the water in your body—the droplets in your lungs, the fluid in your bloodstream. On the inhale, feel yourself breathing your vitality into your body's water; on the exhale, feel your body's water returning the gift to you.

EXERCISE

1. Now place your hands around the water container. Feel the loving connection to water you have just established. Continue to breathe your gifts into the water as you inhale, and to receive the water's gifts as you exhale.

2. If you have a particular physical, emotional, or spiritual concern— a health problem, work challenge, or emotional difficulty— visualize the healing energy that will help transform you and solve the problem. If you are feeling unloved, for example, recall a time that you felt completely loved and breathe that memory into the water. If you are confused about a task at work, recall a state of clarity and breathe that clear mind and sharpened perception into the water. If you have a particular health problem, see your body

and immune system as perfectly whole and healthy, and breathe that vision into the water.

3. You can spend any amount of time on this exercise that seems right to you, from 5 seconds in a crowded restaurant to 15 minutes at home with your week's supply of water. Conclude by connecting to your gratitude to the water for supplying you with life, and to the universe for creating this sharing, loving water.

DRINKING WATER TO IMPROVE YOUR HEALTH

If you want to know the meaning of water, just drink.

—ZEN SAYING

Most people need to drink two liters, or 3.5 pints, of water a day—about seven or eight glasses. The best times to drink are when you get up, before you go to sleep, and between meals, as well as half an hour before eating. Though it may be convenient to drink water with meals, it's actually not a good idea—it can interfere with the digestive properties of your own saliva, which is full of enzymes to help your body break down food into its component nutrients. Some people even suffer indigestion, acid stomach, or nausea from drinking water with their meals. However, drinking before and after eating is excellent for your health, helping to flush out toxins, excess fats, and cholesterol.

Filtered water is ideal because it doesn't contain any of the pollutants and toxins that most tap water now includes. Remember, too, that caffeinated drinks—including coffee, tea, and sodas—are diuretics, which purge your body of water. Nicotine and alcohol also tend to dehydrate you (it's the drying out of the fluids in which your brain floats that causes the painful headache of a hangover). So moderate your intake of caffeine, nicotine, and alcohol—which, as we've also seen, stress your liver and can promote inflammation—and drink extra water to compensate for their dehydrating and toxic effects.

Water is also an excellent weight-loss aid, as Teresa discovered. She began to realize that at times when she thought she was hungry, she was actually thirsty, and she learned to reach for a glass of water rather than a sugary snack. As her relationship to water developed, she also derived some of the comfort and sense of nurture in water that she'd previously found only in her favorite "comfort foods."

Many of my patients have noticed that when they drink water regularly, staying hydrated and keeping their body fluids at a high level, they start to feel less stressed and more calm. I believe that water shares its loving nature with all of us, but there's also a biological reason involved. Many of the body's responses to dehydration are similar to its behavior under stress. By depriving your body of water, you're sending the signal that something is wrong—and your stress hormones react accordingly.

WASHING, BATHING, AND SHOWERING IN THE MATRIX

> The rabbi noticed the servant woman struggling as she drew two heavy buckets of water from the well and lugged them into the house. That night as he washed his hands before the evening meal, he used only a tiny amount of water. A guest noticed what he was doing and asked why he was being so sparing with the water. "Don't you know that it's a blessing to wash our hands, as God has commanded us?" the guest inquired.

"Certainly," the rabbi replied. "But the blessing would be vastly diminished if I were pious at my servant's expense."

—TRADITIONAL JEWISH FOLKTALE, ADAPTED FROM
A TREASURY OF JEWISH FOLKLORE,
EDITED BY NATHAN AUSUBEL

Washing and bathing have always been important in Jewish practice. Traditionally, Jewish men and women are encouraged to visit the *mikveh,* the ritual bath, an ancient kabbalistic technology developed to purify us energetically. Water in the *mikveh* must come from rain, the ocean, or a flowing stream. By immersing ourselves in this water, we become one with the flowing waters of nature.

In Kabbalah, moreover, we assign a numerical value to each Hebrew letter, then add the letters together to find the numerical value of each word. Words with the same numerical value are spiritually linked. I find it significant that the Hebrew letters that spell *mikveh* have the same numerical value as the word *sharing.* Other cultures, too, see bathing as an almost sacred act, particularly when you consider the centuries of human history when water for washing was a significant luxury. Every ounce of water had to be hauled from a well or carried from a stream or spring, or at the very least brought from a pump. No wonder bathing in early societies was often a communal affair, as the ancient Egyptians, Sumerians, Babylonians, Romans, and Arabs created public or religious bathing facilities of various kinds. "Taking the waters" at mineral springs was also a well-established practice conducted over many centuries.

Today, when most of us can get water at the turn of a tap, we have lost our reverence for water, as well as our sense of how this vital element is connected to the running mountain streams or bubbling springs of our planet earth. Nevertheless, washing and bathing continue to be powerful means of accessing the sharing consciousness of water. Washing the hands before eating can be a useful way of focusing our bodies, minds, and spirits on the nourishment we are about to receive, reminding us to open ourselves fully to this conversation with "the fruits of the earth." (For more on eating with full consciousness, see Chapter 5.) Bathing in warm water helps draw the toxins in our bodies to the surface. If we remain in the tub for 20 minutes or more, the cooling water absorbs the toxins and they run down the bathroom drain when we are done. Essential oils, bath salts, and other ingredients can expand the healing power of bathing.

One of the modern pioneers of hydrotherapy was Sebastian Kneipp, a nineteenth-century Dominican priest who believed that the body can heal itself by making use of water and other natural elements. Kneipp developed several specific treatments for various ailments, and today, his name lives on in a popular commercial bath-oil preparation. Here are some adaptations of his suggestions for therapeutic bathing:

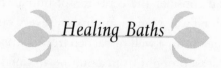

Healing Baths

TO RESTORE ENERGY

1. Fill your tub with cold water, about 60 degrees Fahrenheit (16 degrees Celsius), until the water is 10 inches deep.

2. Remain in the tub, dipping the water over your body, for about a minute.

3. Get out and dry yourself vigorously with a rough towel.

TO RELEASE STRESS

1. Fill your tub halfway with water that is close to body temperature.

2. Gradually add cold water, so that in the course of 15 minutes, the water temperature is 60 degrees Fahrenheit (16 degrees Celsius).

3. Get out and wrap yourself in a large, warm towel. Rest for an hour.

TO RELIEVE PAIN

1. Get into the shower at a comfortably warm temperature and remain there for 2 to 3 minutes.

2. Turn the temperature to cold for up to 3 minutes.

3. Continue to alternate between hot and cold for several turns.

TO RELIEVE PAIN FROM MENSTRUATION, PELVIC INFLAMMATION, OR URINARY TRACT INFECTION

1. Sit in a very hot bath—up to 100 degrees Fahrenheit (23 degrees Celsius)—for about 5 minutes. Do not remain in the hot water any longer than this, as it will have an enervating effect.

2. Get out of the tub and rub yourself with a cooling lotion or rubbing alcohol. Your goal is to cool down quickly but gently from the hot bath.

OR

1. Fill your tub with hot water—about 104 degrees Fahrenheit (25 degrees Celsius)—and add an herbal infusion of juniper berries, rose hips, and horsetail (an herb).

2. Remain in the tub for about 10 minutes.

3. Get out and dry yourself gently with a soft towel.

Of course, the therapeutic effects of all these treatments are magnified a thousandfold if you also allow your new understanding of the sharing, healing properties of water to penetrate your mind and spirit even as you bathe or shower. Remember, water has its own consciousness, giving of itself unconditionally, showing us how to share—and how to become healed through our sharing.

Here's one more ritual, which you can perform every time you wash your hands or take your morning shower:

WASHING TO REFRESH YOUR SPIRIT

1. As you shower or bathe, focus on the healing spirit of the water. Envision it carrying away anything that distresses you, mentally or physically.

2. Feel the water that surrounds you communicating with the fluids inside your body. Experience the love, caring, and sharing that is moving back and forth through your skin, until you are steeped in water's sharing consciousness, inside and outside your body.

3. If you like, create a ritual prayer or use this sample prayer:

> *Water, as I wash with you, I feel your loving, sharing consciousness. I feel you washing away my sorrow and my separateness. I feel you flooding me with joy and connection. I feel myself becoming like you. I feel my own sharing, flowing within me like a fountain.*

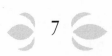

7 LIVING IN THE MATRIX: HEALING YOURSELF "24/7"

TRADITIONAL JEWISH FOLKTALE, ADAPTED FROM *A TREASURY OF JEWISH FOLKLORE*, EDITED BY NATHAN AUSUBEL—

> *Once a miser decided that he was spending far too much money on his horse. "Why should I feed that beast so often?" he asked himself. "Surely, with a little practice, he could be trained not to eat!" Accordingly, the miser began to feed his horse less and less, hoping to train him out of his expensive habits. One day, the miser met a friend who asked him how the experiment was going.*
>
> *"Oh, it was fine for a while," the miser said. "But just when I was on the verge of getting him to eat nothing at all, what do you think happened? The damn horse up and died!"*

MANY of us are tempted to treat ourselves the way the miser in the story treated his horse. We think we can train ourselves to work harder and harder, living with less and less fulfillment, rest, and relaxation. We push ourselves to work from morning till night, we grab our meals on the go, and we consider unscheduled time spent with our loved ones or peaceful times alone luxuries that we can't afford. Then, when we come down with stress-related illnesses or even develop life-threatening disorders, we wonder what went wrong.

I am reminded of Jewelle, a frail young woman with dark circles under her eyes who was suffering from hepatitis B, a debilitating disease that, according to standard medical understanding, can be treated but not cured. When she first came to see me, Jewelle was struggling with the typical hepatitis B symptoms: a reduced appetite, nausea, joint pain, and a persistent fatigue that had lasted for several weeks.

"I feel like I never get a break," Jewelle complained. "These problems are just with me all the time. I feel like I've always been sick and I always will be sick."

To cope with the nausea and build up her system, I helped Jewelle work out her own version of Matrix Nutrition. (For more on food, see Chapter 5, as well as my previous book, *Gut Reactions.*) But I knew that Jewelle needed more than a shift in her approach to food. According to Kabbalah, the liver is the seat of reactive consciousness—and hepatitis is a disease of the liver. Clearly, shifting out of a reactive consciousness was key for Jewelle.

I began by explaining to her the concept of the "kabbalistic day," in which every single moment is viewed as an opportunity for growth and as a chance to experience our higher soul. In such a view, every obstacle that we encounter—from running out of toothpaste to a child's tantrum over breakfast to the bus that makes us late for work—offers us the chance to grow spiritually. The goal is to replace *reactive* responses of the lower soul with *proactive* responses of the Godly soul—the thoughts, feelings, and behavior that we choose from our highest, truest selves. Reactive responses include anger, frustration, envy, fear, and despair, whereas proactive choices of the Godly soul are based in love, compassion, creativity, certainty, and an ultimately optimistic vision of our existence.

I told Jewelle that we all face challenges switching from our lower selves to our Godly selves, no matter how "enlightened" or "spiritual" we are. All of us have buttons that can be pushed, pet peeves, people and situations who just seem to trigger our worst responses.

But Jewelle was unconvinced. "I think I'm already a good person," she told me. "In fact, I know lots of people who behave very badly, and they're not sick at all—so what are you telling me?"

I explained that in Kabbalah, it's not a question of being "good" or "bad." It's a question of each one of us becoming better. A marathon runner doesn't look at a weekend jogger and say, "Well, at least I'm a better runner than *he* is." Instead, she looks at her own athletic challenges and works on them. Does she need to lengthen her stride? Build up her endurance? Work on her final sprint to the finish line? The only way she'll ever grow as an athlete is to identify her limitations and then strive to overcome them.

In exactly the same way, we as human beings are challenged to learn how our buttons get pushed, to understand when we react without thinking and figure out how we act in ways that don't meet our own best standards for good behavior. The point of overcoming these reactive responses is not to become "good people"—although we may indeed become "better people" by doing so. The point is to become more Godly, loving, proactive, creative people—human beings who are truly in control of our own destinies rather than prey to a host of reactive emotions and behaviors.

I suggested to Jewelle that practicing a 24-hour consciousness, an effort to live each moment soulfully, would help her turn toxic feelings of anger, envy, greed, and fear into the healing balm of kindness and compassion. She might do this by consciously choosing to live in her higher Godly soul, even when confronted with obstacles that trigger her lower self and reactive behavior. I suggested that she respond to each difficult situation by thinking of how her higher soul would respond. In so doing, she would not only feel better about herself and her life, she would also be healing her liver and overcoming her disease.

When she finally saw what I was getting at, Jewelle felt more discouraged than ever. "I can barely make it through the day as it is," she snapped. "I don't see how I can expect any more of myself!"

"What if we start with just five minutes," I said as gently as I could. "Just five separate occasions in which you stop, think, and make a different choice?"

Jewelle was still skeptical. But I did my best to convince her that, in my best *medical* opinion, each of those five minutes would be a small but significant boost to her health. Reluctantly, Jewelle agreed to create five proactive moments each day until we had our next appointment the following week.

When I next saw Jewelle, she still seemed skeptical. But she confessed that she'd found herself feeling a bit more energetic that week and she'd actually enjoyed the nutritious food she'd prepared for herself—a significant improvement after many days of nausea and low appetite.

"Those five minutes weren't much," she pointed out. "Most of the time, they were really little things. Like when there was a long line at the grocery store, and I was *so* tired, I wanted to scream. But I forced myself to smile at the person ahead of me and make a joke about it."

"What happened?" I asked.

Jewelle blushed. "Well, actually, he laughed, and then he said, 'You know, you look really tired. Why don't you go ahead of me.'"

As Jewelle continued to get results from her "five proactive moments," she agreed to expand the experiment, adding a few more proactive moments each day. Little by little, she found herself regaining her strength, her energy, and her appetite. She also found herself feeling occasional flashes of serenity and well-being in a way that she hadn't experienced even before her illness.

Jewelle had discovered what Kabbalah makes clear: even tiny shifts can make an enormous difference, infusing your life with a sense of clarity and joy. These small changes accumulate until suddenly we discover that we're making bigger changes, living more and more of our lives as proactive, empowered, and compassionate people.

PAYING ATTENTION TO THE LITTLE THINGS

A wealthy woman once went to see a reknowned yogi and asked for training in spiritual enlightenment. As she sat humbly before the master, she slipped out of her expensive mink coat, letting it slide to the floor in a heap.

The yogi pointed to the coat. "That looks like an expensive coat that cost someone lots of work to make as well as to buy," he said mildly. "Perhaps you ought to care for the coat by hanging it up."

The woman shook her head. "It's really not important—I have lots of coats like that," she said impatiently. "I don't want to waste any more time—let's begin the lesson."

"But many people in the world would be grateful to have that coat," the yogi replied. "Perhaps you might express your gratitude for it by hanging it up properly."

The woman shook her head even more vehemently. "I told you—it doesn't matter," she said. "The coat is only a material possession. I'm here to learn from you about spiritual things."

> Now the yogi shook his head. "I'm afraid the lesson is
> over," he said. "You've already made it clear that there is
> nothing I can teach you."
>
> —TRADITIONAL STORY

How many of us know people who consider themselves "spiritual" or "interested in enlightenment" who nonetheless routinely lose their temper with clerks, browbeat waitresses, or speak rudely to bus drivers? Or what about the person who is unfailingly polite and charming in public while reserving his or her worst behavior for spouse, children, or friends? As the yogi tried to make clear to the woman in the story, proactive behavior is a 24-hour affair. If we're really serious about learning our spiritual lessons, we need to think in terms of taking responsibility for every moment, every action, no matter how small or seemingly insignificant. Kabbalah promises that every moment in which we take that kind of loving care is a moment that boosts our physical as well as our spiritual health.

Numerous scientific studies back up the kabbalists' claims. One researcher studied over one thousand patients who survived a myocardial infarction (heart attack), trying to see whether they could alter the Type A behavior that had presumably worsened their disease. Type A behavior is the kind of outer-directed anger—what kabbalists would call reactive behavior—in which the patients might yell at a taxi driver or a red light while stuck in traffic, rather than choosing a more calm and controlled response. This researcher discovered that more than 98 percent of the cardiac patients he studied did indeed exhibit this type of hostility and time-urgency. He went on to arrange different treatment for the patients:

- 300 patients received information on diet, exercise, and weight control—the standard advice given to those who've had a myocardial infarction.

- 600 patients received this type of advice plus advice on changing to another type of behavior.

- 150 patients received no counseling at all.

After five years, the researcher found that the rate of recurrence of nonfatal myocardial infarctions was lowest among those who had learned to change their behavior—three times lower, in fact, than among those who had received only the standard advice, and four times lower than among those who had received no advice. Clearly, shifting from reactive to proactive responses was good for those heart patients' health.

Of course, some of the benefits of this new approach were biological. The new, calmer behavior released fewer stress hormones, which in turn caused less inflammation, was less likely to spur an increase in blood pressure, and generally made for less strain on the heart. But I would argue that the biological benefits also came from a spiritual source: that feeling serene and in control of our own behavior is simply good for our physical selves.

Numerous recent studies showing a connection between chronic depression and heart disease support this conclusion. In 1996, for example, the journal *Circulation* published the results of a twenty-seven-year study establishing a clear link between depression and the risk of having a heart attack. This study tracked 730 men and women in Denmark who were evaluated in 1964 and 1974 for signs of depression. Those who ranked high on the scale of depressive symptoms were found to have a 70 percent increased risk of heart attack. Indeed, those who had a high number of depressive symptoms when the study began were 60 percent more likely to die early from any cause.

A similar Finnish study of nearly 1,200 men measured subjects for depression with questions about general apathy, happiness, personal worth, concerns about failing health, sleep disturbances, sensitivity to criticism, and lack of positive social interaction. The men also underwent ultrasound evaluations of their carotid arteries to test for atherosclerosis. Although depression itself did not appear to increase the risk of atherosclerosis in the Finnish study, it did magnify other cardiovascular risk factors. For example, depressed smokers had almost three times as much arterial blockage as smokers who were not depressed, while depressed patients with high levels of LDL cholesterol had nearly twice the arterial narrowing as their nondepressed counterparts. Among those with high levels of fibrinogen—a component in the blood-clotting process that is associated with atherosclerosis—the degree of arterial blockage was four times greater among depressed patients than among those who were not depressed.

A study at the Montreal Heart Institute found even more direct links between depression and heart disease. In 1993, N. Frasure-Smith, F. Lesperance, and M. Talasic examined 222 survivors of major heart attacks. The researchers found that survivors suffering from major depression risked dying within six months of the attack at a rate that was three to four times greater than their nondepressed counterparts, even after all other factors associated with heart disease had been adjusted for. In other words, depression is as great a mortality risk as the degree of actual damage to the heart.

Interestingly, in the Montreal study, depression was associated with a lack of close friends. The notion that isolation is harmful is further supported by Kenneth R. Pelletier, Ph.D., in his book *Sound Mind, Sound Body,* in which Pelletier argues that optimal health is rooted in a positive, purposeful life orientation, and that people who feel a strong sense of belonging and connection with others are better able to withstand stress, have fewer illnesses, and live longer. Pelletier also shows that people with altruistic beliefs and behavior are remarkably resistant to chronic disease.

Moreover, Pelletier discovered that overcoming childhood traumas and other difficulties seemed to lead the people he studied to develop compassion, commitment—and resistance to physical illness. This bears out the kabbalistic notion that the process of overcoming a challenge is more important than the "absolute" sense of a person's moral standing. It's the effort to get better that matters, not where you start or where you end up.

Finally, Pelletier found, increased life expectancy and improved health are both associated with a drive toward a deeper sense of meaning and purpose in life. In kabbalistic terms, compassionate connections with others literally help us to expand our vessel— the metaphor for the self—making us more able to withstand stress and hardship without physical difficulties.

Pelletier's work is eloquently echoed by psychologist Robert Ornstein and physician David Sobel, the Stanford University professor of neurobiology and Kaiser-Permanente Health System executive who co-wrote *The Healing Brain.* In that groundbreaking book, the authors comment, "The sense of connectedness and responsibility, whether it be to people, pets, or plants, seems to draw us out of ourselves and link us to a larger world. The predisposition to communicate with others, to bond, appears to be vital to our health."

THE HEALING POWER OF DOING GOOD

> A rich man was dying because, although his fever had gone
> up very high, he was unable to sweat. His doctor had tried
> every possible means to induce perspiration, but to no avail.
>
> Finally, convinced he was going to die, the rich man sent
> for the rabbi and arranged to make over a large portion of
> his wealth to the local synagogue and its many charities. He
> signed the affidavit, and the rabbi began to leave the room.
> "Hold on, rabbi!" the rich man called out abruptly. "All of a
> sudden—I'm sweating!"
>
> —TRADITIONAL JEWISH JOKE, ADAPTED FROM *A TREASURY OF*
> *JEWISH FOLKLORE*, EDITED BY NATHAN AUSUBEL

The joke here, of course, is that only the prospect of losing money can cause the rich man to sweat. But I like the way this story makes clear—albeit in a humorous way—that compassion for others and charitable behavior really do lead to greater health.

This notion is more seriously expressed in a book by Allan Luks, *The Healing Power of Doing Good: The Health and Spiritual Benefits of Helping Others.* Luks, a former Peace Corps worker, community-action lawyer in East Harlem, and head of the Institute for the Advancement of Health, surveyed over 3,000 volunteers to discover that when people help others, those who offer assistance often experience a "helper's high"—a sudden rush of warmth, good feelings, and increased energy, followed by a longer-lasting sense of calm, well-being, and self-worth. Students of Matrix Healing won't be surprised to learn that people who frequently experience "helper's high" also report generally high levels of overall health.

Luks advises people to help strangers—people to whom we feel no obvious sense of obligation—as well as giving of ourselves to family and friends. Giving out of a sense of duty, he points out, is less likely to lead to a helper's high, and from a Matrix Healing perspective, less likely to improve our health.

Luks also suggests that we let go of results and focus on the process of helping and the feelings of closeness, warmth, and satisfaction that it engenders. As a Matrix Healer, I would say that looking at the results of our helpfulness is really a form of ego, in which we seek to feel good about our own achievements rather than to genuinely empathize with another person in need. The best way to improve our health is by focusing on the needs and well-being of others.

When Jewelle and I discussed the role of empathy in her life, she once again expressed despair. "I'm just not that kind of person," she told me. "I try my best to do the right thing—but it's not really an emotional thing with me."

I reassured Jewelle that empathy and compassion can be learned and developed. The important thing is to practice becoming proactive at every opportunity, to interrupt our reactive behavior so that we have a chance to look at things from another person's point of view or simply to respond emotionally to his or her predicament. I believe that something deep inside our cells responds positively when we feel our own humanity, when we are stirred to put aside the lens of ego that clouds our vision, when we experience the compassion that is the truest expression of our souls.

LISTENING TO OUR HEARTS

> I shall give you a new heart, and I shall put a new spirit
> within you. I shall remove the heart of stone from within
> your flesh, and give you a heart of flesh.
>
> —EZEKIEL 36:26

One of the things I try to convey to my patients is the profound truth of this quote from Ezekiel. Once you begin to live in the Matrix, you feel as though your heart literally comes alive and your spirit is restored. You begin to understand that the heart has its own wisdom and that literally, on a biological level, the brain is meant to listen to the heart.

Recent embryological research has shown that this heart-brain connection begins in the womb, when the tiny human embryo is first formed. At this origin of human development, the heart and the brain are side by side. As the embryo develops, a physical separation occurs but the biological connection remains. Through both connective neurological tissue and electromagnetic interconnections, the brain and heart continue their conversation. Neurotransmitters—those biochemical substances that transmit commands to the body's muscles, organs, and glands—are found in both the brain and the heart, establishing a far deeper and more complicated connection between these two organs than I was ever taught about in medical school.

Thus, contrary to prevailing medical wisdom, it seems that the heart exerts at least as much control over the brain as the brain maintains over the heart. As Paul Pearsall writes in his book *The Heart's Code,* recent studies by Dr. John and Beatrice Lacey at National Institute of Mental Health have turned up direct evidence that the heart requests a continual environmental update from the brain in order to organize the body's energy. Through neurohormones, the heart requests information and then acts upon that information to regulate the body's activity.

The Laceys discovered that the heart also produces a hormone known as Atrial Naturetic Factor (ANF) peptide, which is released into the bloodstream each time the muscles of the atrium contract. This ANF peptide sends messages to the brain, immune system, hypothalamus, thalamus, pituitary, and pineal gland. The hypothalamus helps regulate stress and other emotional states; the thalamus and pituitary are involved with the brain's limbic system of emotions, memory, and learning; and the pineal gland helps to regulate the sleep/wake cycle, the aging process, and our energy levels throughout the day. Thus, the heart is literally participating in a body-wide conversation with the brain—truly, a heart of flesh that is very far from the mechanistic model I was presented with in medical school.

Further research into the heart's intelligence is being conducted at the Institute of Heart Medicine (IHM). For example, in a 1992 study, two groups of rabbits were fed the same high-fat diet. One group, however, was shown loving behavior by the researchers, who handled the rabbits gently, spoke to them affectionately, and petted them. Another group was given standard treatment. The "loved" rabbits developed significantly less atherosclerosis than their "unloved" counterparts, suggesting the healing power of love.

The rabbits were only the recipients of love. What happens when you are the one to feel love and compassion for another person?

As we saw in Chapter 1, Harvard University researcher A. Thomas McLelland found that when people experience compassion, their salivary IgA levels go up. IgA is an antibody that is generally considered the immune system's first line of defense.

McClelland showed people a film of someone behaving compassionately and then measured the viewers' IgA levels. He found that even those subjects who reported no consciously positive response to the film experienced an immunological boost.

Researchers at the Institute of Heart Medicine have replicated McClelland's work and then built on it in two interesting ways. First, they discovered that when research subjects generated their own experiences of compassion, rather than simply responding to a movie, their IgA levels went up even further. They also found that what I would call reactive behavior—experiences of anger and frustration—suppressed the immune system, both when new occasions for anger emerged and when research subjects were rehashing an old experience that had made them angry. Clearly, proactive states of compassion and love are good for your health, while anger, frustration, and other types of reactive behavior are unhealthy.

Finally, IHM researchers have also discovered that compassion boosts your levels of DHEA, a growth hormone with antiaging properties. IHM studies showed that some subjects achieved a 100 percent increase in DHEA levels after only one month of practicing compassionate responses. By the same token, cortisol—the stress hormone associated with inflammation and weight gain—decreases in response to compassionate feelings. Apparently, just five minutes of feeling compassion for another person enhances your immune system, whereas five minutes of anger or anxiety suppresses it for hours.

HEALING AND THE HUMAN CONNECTION

> The quality of mercy is not strain'd.
>
> It droppeth as the gentle rain from heaven
>
> Upon the place beneath; it is twice blest:

It blesseth him that gives and him that takes. . . .

It is an attribute to God himself. . . .

—WILLIAM SHAKESPEARE, *THE MERCHANT OF VENICE*

We've seen that compassionate behavior—whether it is given or received—helps boost the immune system and enhances your general health. These findings are consistent with the numerous studies showing that patients benefit from social support. Isolated patients tend to be less healthy than those with a wide, supportive network of friends, family, or neighbors.

Although the connection between isolation and ill health is well known, some researchers have viewed this in purely practical terms. Social support is helpful, they argue, not because of any spiritual benefit so much as because it means that people are likely to get the medical and therapeutic help they need.

While this is undoubtedly true, I would argue that a deeper process is at work: the powerful effects of the cycle of giving, receiving, and sharing—a cycle that benefits both the person who gives and the one who receives. This mutual benefit is evident in numerous studies showing that those who do regular volunteer work or who give in other ways often have better health outcomes than their nonvolunteering counterparts, even if the nonvolunteers score higher on the social contact scale and have better personal support networks.

Apparently, diversity of social contacts is also a health factor—in my view, because the wider your set of friends and acquaintances, the more your Vessel expands to admit new possibilities and the healthier you become as a result. One study in which subjects were deliberately injected with a virus and then monitored to see whether they became sick found that the more diverse people's social relationships were—including friends, co-workers, and relatives—the less likely they were to catch colds. People who had contact at least once every two weeks with six or more types of relationships fought off colds best and had less than one-quarter the risk of getting sick when compared with those who had only one, two, or three types of relationships. What seemed to matter in this study was not the total number of relationships but rather their diversity. People who had a large number of friends, but only from work, for example, tended to be less healthy than those who had fewer friends but from different walks of life.

When Jewelle learned about these studies, she began to seriously rethink several decisions she had made in her life. She had always considered that friends and a social life should take second place to establishing financial security. Although she was happily married to a devoted husband, she realized that they had both allowed their social circle to narrow to just the two of them, believing that friends were a luxury that could come after they'd moved up the career ladder.

The perspective I shared with her, however, led her to realize that her narrow focus on financial security was actually injuring her health. "I thought that having this disease meant I needed to cut back," Jewelle told me. "But from what you're telling me, I need to reach out more."

Although she still felt weak and shaky from her hepatitis B symptoms, Jewelle began to reach out to those around her. In addition to her daily "proactive minutes," she volunteered to make weekly visits to a local nursing home. She became close to a few residents in particular, reading to them and talking with them each week. To her surprise—but not to mine—Jewelle began to find that instead of draining her, each visit generated more energy, which replenished both her body and her spirit. She also reestablished some old friendships she had allowed to fade and again discovered that the social activities helped to restore her health and spirits. Through these new efforts, Jewelle began to see that the development of "heart's wisdom" and proactivity is a lifelong process that takes place, not all at once, but every minute of every day, in the face of new challenges and difficulties—but always with the promise of new rewards.

OVERCOMING ANGER

One afternoon, as the Rabbi of Vizhnitz was supervising the preparation of matzohs for Passover, he noticed that one of his students had shouted at one of the women who was rolling out the matzoh dough.

"My son, you must never shout," he told his student.

"But rabbi," said the student, "even the slightest trace of leavened bread is forbidden."

The rabbi shook his head. "Of course the slightest trace of leavened bread is forbidden," he said. "But the slightest trace of rage is an even greater transgression."

—ADAPTED WITH PERMISSION FROM
RABBI ABRAHAM J. TWERSKI, M.D., *NOT JUST STORIES*,
ARTSCROLL/MESORAH PUBLICATIONS

Over the past few decades, scientists have begun to assert that too much anger can be harmful to our health. The angry Type A personality, for example, is considered to be at risk for heart disease. In addition to being angry and/or hostile, Type A people are typically extremely competitive, aggressive, and achievement-oriented. They experience enormous time-urgency, speak explosively, and frequently express hostility. Dr. Karen A. Matthews, a renowned psychosocial epidemiologist and investigator into the

Type A personality, working with colleagues from the Universities of Michigan and North Carolina, has concluded that the Type A personality is also characterized by a drive to accumulate wealth and possessions beyond his or her immediate needs.

Rather than viewing the Type A personality as an emotional syndrome, I would suggest we consider it a spiritual problem. The anger, competitiveness, and aggression represent reactive behavior, and the greed for extra possessions speaks to a lack of certainty in the world's abundance and generosity.

It behooves us to look closely at how and why Type A personalities operate, since according to the latest scientific studies, psychosocial and emotional factors are the most significant risk factors in the development of heart disease, as well as the most significant factors in the prediction of outcome—far more than the traditional risk factors of smoking, cholesterol, and hypertension. Apparently, it would do patients more good to learn how to deal with anger, depression, and hostility than to quit smoking, lower cholesterol, or decrease blood pressure.

For example, typically, one-third of patients who undergo angioplasty—a procedure that opens blocked arteries—must undergo a second procedure within six months. Yet a study published in the *Mayo Clinic Proceedings* of 1996 reveals that patients who tend to be angry or hostile are more than twice as likely to undergo the repeated procedure than patients without huge stores of anger. Clearly, anger is a significant risk factor for arterial blockage.

Likewise, anxiety associated with hostility and anger has been found to be one of the strongest risk factors for sudden cardiac arrest—up to six times more dangerous than cigarettes or other known risk factors. Clearly, doctors would do well to consider ways of helping their patients overcome anger, anxiety, and other forms of reactive behavior.

Very few physicians have done this, but Redford Williams, M.D., is one who has. Williams is director of behavioral research at Duke University Medical Center, professor of psychiatry, and associate professor of medicine. He is also the author of several books on anger, including *The Trusting Heart,* an in-depth look at research on the connection between hostility and disease, and *Anger Kills: Seventeen Strategies for Controlling the Hostility That Can Harm Your Health,* written with Virginia Williams, a compendium of practical ways for diffusing anger, hostility, and cynicism.

Although many experts have advised "talking out" one's anger, expressing it fully in order to "release" it, Williams shows that this approach is actually more likely to increase anger than to defuse it. Sometimes, of course, it's important to express our anger, telling a supervisor, competitor, or even a loved one that he or she has crossed a boundary. But even such expressions are often best done after the anger has passed, when we can speak with compassion and listen attentively to the response. Meanwhile, Williams suggests, it's healthier—both psychologically and physically—to defuse anger in other ways: reasoning with oneself, learning forgiveness, caring for a pet.

Indeed, the Institute of Heart Math conducted a small but powerful experiment in the health benefits of such care. They were monitoring a number of subjects for heart rate variability (HRV), an important factor in cardiovascular problems. One of their subjects, a construction worker, frequently got angry and upset at work, causing marked changes in his HRV. Yet when this same man began caring for a rabbit—which he eventually even took to work with him—his HRV pattern improved.

As a physician, I'm glad to see that Williams and the Institute of Heart Math are taking up this issue, and I hope other doctors go on to share this approach with their patients. But from my perspective as a Matrix Healer, I would again add a spiritual dimension. In my view, the most powerful antidote to anger and other reactive behavior is the deeper understanding that anger takes away our proactive, God-like ability to choose our own responses. Losing our tempers or descending into cynicism replaces this empowered, God-like self with a reactive being at the mercy of his or her emotions.

Another powerful antidote to anger is a wider view of the world, which leads to a deeper experience of compassion. Once we see ourselves as part of the true "ecology of spirit," which I outline in Chapter 9, we find our emotions shifting accordingly. It's far more difficult being angry at others when we see them as deeply connected to ourselves.

A deeper connection with nature also mitigates against anger, as researcher R. Kaplan found in a 1973 study. When Kaplan asked 1,000 office workers about what they saw from their office windows, he discovered that workers who had views of nature—trees, flowers, and the like—reported double the job satisfaction of workers who saw only buildings and human-made objects. The workers who could see some aspect of nature felt less frustrated and more patient, found their jobs more satisfying, expressed more enthusiasm during their day, and reported a greater sense of well-being and better health. Well-being and health were also associated with access to nature near the workers' homes.

Likewise, Roger Ulrich found that surgical patients with a view of a park recovered more quickly, needed fewer pain medications, and were discharged earlier than patients in the more typical hospital room without a view. Evidently, being connected to nature increases our sense of wholeness. Restoring our sense of intimacy with nature makes us feel as though we are at home in the world, a secure and peaceful feeling that mitigates against anger and helps create health.

These studies make eminent sense to me because I've long

believed that one of the greatest gifts we have—and one of the most important factors in staying healthy—is our natural sense of wonder. How do we lose our initial sense of awe and pleasure at the beauty in the natural world? Those of us who have kept that sense of wonder alive have taken a giant step on the road of health. To quote Albert Einstein, "The fairest thing we can experience is the mysterious. It is the fundamental emotion that stands at the cradle of true art and true science. He who does not know it and can no longer wonder, no longer feel amazement, is as good as dead—a snuffed-out candle."

What I personally see when I look at nature is a magnificent design that we humans can understand imperfectly at best. To me, therefore, the natural world evokes profound humility— a humility that mitigates against the Type A responses of anger and urgency and toward a sense of acceptance and calm that alleviates stress, lowers blood pressure, and generally helps us find a harmonious balance, within ourselves and in our lives.

SHIFTING FROM A REACTIVE TO A PROACTIVE CONSCIOUSNESS

> During a space flight, the psyche of each astronaut is reshaped. Having seen the sun, the stars, and our planet, you become more full of life, softer. You begin to look at all living things with greater trepidation, and you begin to be more kind and patient with the people around you.
>
> —BORIS VOLYNOV, SOVIET COSMONAUT

Here are some of the exercises I shared with Jewelle as she sought to become more proactive throughout her day. Although initially, Jewelle had seen the idea of "24-hour consciousness" as an intolerable burden, she came to enjoy the notion that every moment of every day offers us new opportunities for empowering ourselves and making creative, authentic, and fulfilling choices.

WAKING UP

Instead of hitting the snooze button or heading for the bathroom in a daze, try doing a simple stretching exercise while you're still lying in bed.

1. Throughout this exercise, remain aware of your body. Your goal is to focus entirely on how you feel physically.

2. Lie on your back with your arms extended loosely downward, one on each side. If necessary, put a pillow under the small of your back so you can lie stretched out full-length.

3. Very, very gently, elongate your neck. Think of yourself as adding two inches to your height. (If you feel any twinges or soreness, stop immediately.)

4. Stretch your shoulders by moving them downward. Keep the image in your mind of adding inches to your height. As your shoulders move downward, imagine your head floating higher.

5. Stretch your arms. Move your mind down through your upper arms, elbows, lower arms, wrists, palms, and then throughout your fingers.

6. Stretch your torso. Again, feel yourself getting longer, taller. As you stretch your torso, gently raise your arms—keeping them flat against the bed—until your arms are above your head.

7. Stretch your hips, extending them downward as your arms reach upward. All parts of your body should be lying flat against the bed.

8. As you continue to stretch your arms upward, continue to stretch downward through your thighs, knees, calves, ankles, feet, toes.

9. Extend your entire body, from the crown of your head down through your toes, as your arms reach upward. Stretch as slowly as you can, reaching as far as you can in both directions, with your mind entirely focused on your physical sensations.

10. Hold your stretch for 30 seconds, breathing in and out slowly and deeply. Allow yourself to take pleasure in your physical health and in your awareness of the present moment.

11. Relax, roll over gently, and get out of bed. During the day, when you feel tense or frustrated, allow your mind to recall your physical pleasure.

GETTING DRESSED

Use your moment of selecting clothes for the day as a chance to make new choices for yourself—to re-create yourself. Ask yourself these questions as you get dressed:

1. **What part of my personality would I like to express today?** Consider choosing at least one item of clothing to bring out a part of your personality that you don't usually allow yourself to express. If you're a responsible executive, can you demonstrate a bit of your artistic side? If you're usually straitlaced, can you add some sexuality to the picture? If you're a carefree, artistic type, how about showing the part of you that is determined and responsible?

2. **What will bring me joy today?** Is there a piece of clothing or jewelry whose colors bring you pleasure? Whose texture you enjoy? That reminds you of someone you care about? As you choose that piece of apparel, think of yourself as choosing all the

joy that goes with it—and then allow yourself to carry those feelings with you throughout the day.

Remember, anytime you challenge yourself—even with something as simple as your wardrobe—you're boosting your immune system and improving your health. And any choices you make—even the apparently small ones of choosing your clothes—strengthen your choice-making capacity for larger issues.

DURING THE DAY

At a moment when you're feeling tired, bored, or frustrated, make a conscious effort to shift your mood.

1. Focus on something in your life that brings you joy—an aspect of your work, your life partner, a child, the sight of the tree outside your window.

2. Find a way to make a joke.

3. Take a break.

4. Do something that gives you pleasure—drinking a cup of tea, taking a brisk walk, calling a friend, e-mailing a loved one.

5. Stop and check in with your body. Do a breathing exercise, or a stretching exercise. Or simply stop, shut your eyes, and become aware of where you are and how you feel.

6. Shift perspective. Is what's upsetting you really so terrible? Is there another way to respond? Is there someone you can ask for help? Is there some way to help yourself?

7. Acknowledge your feelings. If you're genuinely angry, sorrowful, scared, frustrated, worried, or simply "down in the dumps,"

sometimes saying, "Right now I feel———" can help your emotions seem less overwhelming. You may find yourself able to experience the emotion without feeling swamped by it.

As we've discussed, shifting your mood can literally boost your immune system and help combat a whole host of stress-related illnesses. Every time you interrupt an automatic response to choose a conscious, loving action over a hasty reaction, you've given yourself a dose of "spontaneous remission"—a healthy, life-giving moment, whether you are sick or well.

A FOUR-STEP PROGRAM FOR BECOMING PROACTIVE

Who is a hero? He who becomes master over his passions.
—THE ETHICS OF THE FATHERS

Numerous studies show that stress of various types can adversely affect our immune systems, leading researchers Robert Ornstein and David Sobel to ask whether we can voluntarily alter our immune function. In a review of twenty-two studies, Ornstein and Sobel, authors of *The Healing Brain,* found that mental interventions or self-regulation techniques can significantly change our ability to withstand disease and various disorders. The studies under review considered a variety of techniques, including relaxation, guided imagery, music therapy, self-hypnosis, meditation, and biofeedback. Eighteen of the twenty-two studies revealed positive changes on various immunological measures based on the use of one or more mind therapies.

Likewise, Karen Olness and her colleagues conducted a number of their own studies showing that, with practice, people could learn to control various aspects of immune function. One method they used was to teach patients to enter into a relaxed state and then to engage in guided imagery and visualization. One set of subjects visualized their neutrophils—immune cells—as Ping-Pong balls with honey oozing out onto their surface, causing them to stick to everything they came in contact with. According to Olness and her colleagues, these subjects' neutrophils did indeed function as though they had increased stickiness.

Another approach to modifying our consciousness is suggested by Jeffrey M. Schwartz, M.D., in his book *The Mind and the Brain,* which he co-authored with Sharon Begley. Schwartz, a UCLA psychiatrist and a specialist in obsessive-compulsive disorder (OCD), created a four-step program to help his OCD patients distinguish between their minds and their brains. In Schwartz's view, the OCD patients' brains were characterized by "faulty wiring"—neurochemical problems that caused the patients to receive repeated messages requiring them to undertake absurd repetitive behavior. However, if the patients could learn to see that they possessed a mind—a self—that was greater than their physical brains, they could rely on that other self and overcome their brains' problematic demands. This process, Schwartz believed, literally changed his patients' brain chemistry and could potentially be adapted to other syndromes, such as Tourette's, stammering, and depression.

I believe Schwartz's approach also works for Matrix Healers who want to become more proactive. Adapting his methodology, I would offer the following four-step program for overcoming reactive behavior:

1. **Relabel the reactive impulse.** When you experience the wish to lash out in anger, or the impulse to feel envious, or even

the desire to eat a type of food you know is unhealthy for you, label your impulse accordingly. Say to yourself, "This isn't what I truly desire, it's simply an impulse of my reactive nature."

2. **Reattribute the impulse.** Tell yourself where this impulse comes from, portraying your reactive nature as specifically as you can. You might reattribute the impulse in psychological terms: "I only have this wish because I am feeling lonely." "I only feel envious because I'm not in touch with the world's abundance." "I only feel like eating because I am angry." Or you might visualize your reactive nature as the force of gravity, or the force of entropy, pulling you down or engaging you in the process of decay. However you think of your own reactive impulse, be clear that it is just that—an impulse of your reactive nature, and not the sum total of your desires.

3. **Refocus.** Make a conscious effort to replace the impulse with something else. Say, "Instead of envying that person, I will focus on the things I admire about him," or "I'll think about someone I love without envy," or even, "I'll think about all the things I have to be proud of." Or recall a time when you felt love and compassion, and bring the emotions that accompanied those responses back into your consciousness. You might even take specific action—calling a friend in need, reaching out for help and comfort, or taking a creative step to improve your own life.

4. **Revalue the reactive impulse.** How many of us, when we feel depressed, anxious, or lonely, consider those impulses to be of immense significance, reflecting some dire reality that we must discover and change? What if instead, like Schwartz's patients, we simply decided that these reactive responses— along with our feelings of anger, greed, envy, and insecurity— were artifacts of our reactive nature, illusions that are no more useful in helping us navigate reality than the insistent

rituals of an OCD patient? Step 4, then, is to remind yourself
that your initial impulse was meaningless—simply a trick of
your reactive nature to drag you down or pull you apart.
What is meaningful is the love you feel and the compassion
you experience. Your reactive impulses masquerade as your
true self, but they're really just noise—"a tale told by an idiot;
full of sound and fury, signifying nothing," to quote
Shakespeare once again.

Remember that the kabbalists refer to the force of reactivity as
Satan, a code word not for an actual devil but for the gravity or
entropy that drags us down and tricks us into thinking that we're
nothing more than the sum of our impulses. The words of Rabbi
Berg bear repeating: "Satan's greatest triumph is convincing us
that he doesn't exist." In other words, notice how frequently
we're tempted to see our reactive impulses as coming from our
true self rather than as tricks of Satan to pull us away from the
path of true empowerment. Next time you feel a reactive
impulse coming on, try this four-step program. If nothing else, it
will help you slow down and think through who you really are
and what you really want—and that in itself may be enough to
frustrate your reactive nature.

THE SABBATH: A DAY OF ABUNDANCE

Blessed are you, O Lord, our God, King of the world, who
has given me all my requirements.

—KABBALISTIC PRAYER

As we consider the notion of 24-hour consciousness, we can't forget the most special day of the week: the Sabbath, or *Shabat*. Begin-

ning on Friday evening and ending at sundown on Saturday, this Sabbath day is endowed with a special energy that redefines life as inherently spiritual. From this vantage point, we are already healed, and we can begin to taste the abundance of life. Indeed, according to Kabbalah, when life is viewed this way, its spiritual essence is unlimited and bountiful, and the seventh day is so spiritually powerful that it is considered a day when we are healed.

As we saw in Chapter 1, physicists believe that there are particular moments—choice points—when parallel universes become uniquely available. *Shabat* is one of those choice points, at which we draw unusually near to the Matrix and its supply of endless healing energy. Thus, meditating for even a short time on this special day on the worldview *Shabat* offers us can have remarkably powerful Healing effects.

My patient Annette is a case in point. A lively, energetic woman in her fifties, Annette felt that she had always lived life to the fullest. She had a husband whom she loved, three children she adored, and a hitherto satisfying career as a learning-disabilities specialist in a private school. Yet when she hit menopause, Annette was thrown for a loop. Suddenly, she was plagued by a host of symptoms, including persistent fatigue and depression.

As always with my patients, I helped Annette find nutritional supplements and dietary suggestions to respond to her condition, and she also started taking plant-based estrogen (which I find has fewer side effects than standard hormone replacement therapy). Up until now, Annette had been operating full-speed and nonstop, every day of her life. When I asked her to describe a typical week, she shook her head, laughed ruefully, and launched into a daunting list of activities that included a demanding workday, the upkeep of her three-bedroom home, helping her children with their homework, and ferrying them back and forth to music lessons, play dates with friends, after-school theater programs, soccer matches, baseball games, and doctors' appointments. Although her husband was an active participant in their household life, sharing in the cooking, housework, and child care, he, too, had a demanding job, as a freelance computer consultant, which involved working long hours in his home office at all times of the day and night.

"Annette," I said to her frankly, "I think you and your family could all use some time to just do *nothing*."

She laughed again. "Sounds good to me," she said. "But when?"

I told Annette about the kabbalistic concept of the Sabbath as a day for letting go of responsibilities, for trusting in the bounty of life that emanates from the spiritual source of the day. Why work and be stressed if we truly grasp this worldview?

Annette began to slow down on the seventh day and to enjoy the new worldview that the Sabbath offered her. On Saturdays, she started to take more time to meditate, to take walks, and to be with her family. She began to sense that her soul was finally shining through. She gradually came to feel like her old self again, with a renewed sense of purpose and a kind of tranquillity that, she said, belonged to a "new self." "When you're used to pushing yourself so hard, it can actually be kind of painful to stop," she told me several months later. "I think it's taken time for all of us to see the value in doing *nothing*. But believe me, I see it now!"

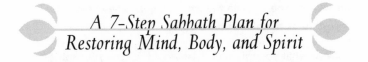

A 7-Step Sabbath Plan for Restoring Mind, Body, and Spirit

1. Remember that the Sabbath begins at sundown Friday night and ends at sundown Saturday night. Find out when sundown will be, and start your Sabbath by paying attention to the setting sun. Notice how your energy shifts as the light changes. Pay attention to the subtle changes in your body in response to the ending of the day and the coming of the night. Tune in to the changes in the world around you as the daylight ends and the twilight begins. Find the relationship between your own biorhythms and the rhythms of the people, animals, trees, and plants around you.

2. Turn off the phone and put a "not available" message on the answering machine. Turn your computer off and keep it off! Turn off any other means of communication with the outside world—fax, radio, television. Remember, this is a day for turning within, for focusing on yourself and your inner resources, for connecting with all of life. If you live with a partner, with roommates, or with children, it can be a day for focusing on one another. Find ways of enjoying your own or each other's company.

3. Arrange to shop and pay your bills on a different day. Save the housework for another time. Today you're finding out what it feels like when you already have everything you need.

4. Explore ways of getting where you want to go that don't involve machinery. Where can you go by foot? Are you able to ride a bike somewhere? Roller skate? Skateboard? Pay attention to the way your world changes when you are focused on where you are, not on where you want to go. Notice how different it feels to get somewhere under your own steam, rather than being carried. Find

out what happens when the *way* you get somewhere is as important as the place you're going.

5. Think of what you might do that would restore your spirit— observing nature, enjoying song, truly experiencing others, contemplating the depths that life can offer.

6. Explore other Sabbath options for your family. Are there ways that your family can be part of a community *as* a family? Are there things you can do together that don't involve machinery or spending money? (Here's a list to get you started: visiting a park together; going on a bike trip or a walk; visiting neighbors or having them visit you.)

7. Contemplate this ancient and yet pioneering worldview that the Sabbath offers. Think of how it transforms the way we see ourselves and our world.

Even if you don't choose to set aside *Shabat* as a healing day, I urge you to take just five minutes of the seventh day—Friday evening or Saturday before sundown—to meditate on our abundant spiritual universe and the possibilities it offers. This is the sense in which the Sabbath is a day of rest, because if the universe has already provided us with perfect health, happiness, and abundance, why should we do anything *but* rest? Once you begin tapping into the special energies of the seventh day, you'll find them a powerful aid to your own self-healing.

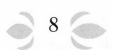

8 PRAYER AND MEDITATION: MATRIX HEALING SOFTWARE THAT CAN CHANGE YOUR LIFE

TRADITIONAL JEWISH FOLKTALE, ADAPTED FROM *A TREASURY OF JEWISH FOLKLORE*, EDITED BY NATHAN AUSUBEL—

The local rabbi was very close to death. His congregation declared a day of fasting, to induce God to save his life. All the Jews in the village gathered to pray in the synagogue, even as the town drunkard went off to the tavern for a brandy. Another Jew saw the drunkard on his way and said, "Hey, today is a fast day! Everyone is going to the synagogue to pray for the rabbi!"

So the drunkard went to the synagogue, too, where he prayed, "Dear God, please save our rabbi's life so I can drink my brandy!"

Miraculously, the rabbi recovered. Later, he told his congregation, "I was saved by our town drunkard. Of all of you, he was the one whose request was heard by God, for he put his whole heart and soul into his prayer!"

I'M especially fond of the story of the drunkard's prayer because it's such a spectacular reminder of what Kabbalah tries to teach us. Our goal is not to become perfect (the drunkard was far from that!) or even to become better than our fellow humans (the drunkard was not that, either). Rather, our goal is to overcome our own reactive natures. From a Matrix Healing perspective, the drunkard's prayer had power because he was able, even for a short time, to resist his will to drink in order to help save the rabbi. The power of his prayer lay in his sincerity, certainty, and compassion.

Prayer is an opportunity to return to our roots, our spiritual essence, our inner point of origin, which is buried deep within our unconscious. According to the Midrash, prayer is a return from fantasy to reality. In reality, the Midrash teaches, the entire world—the whole animal, vegetable, and mineral kingdom—is in a constant state of song, and when we touch this inner divine point of origin, we begin to hear this song.

In prayer, according to Kabbalah, we bind with the divine, becoming one with the Author and becoming Co-Creators of Destiny. Prayer, the Zohar says, is the spine of our spiritual body—our very essence. Indeed, the Mishnah and the Talmud use as a synonym for the human being the Hebrew word mav'eh, which is derived from a Hebrew word that means "to pray." Thus, the Talmud defines the human being as the creature who prays.

In order to make use of this extraordinary power, however, whether for healing or for any other purpose, we need to know the technology of prayer—a healing software that Kabbalah explains in detail, and that I'm now making available here.

My patient Malcolm was especially interested in the connection between kabbalistic prayer and certainty. Malcolm was a tall, quiet man in his mid-thirties who had already achieved considerable success with a number of commercial ventures. Yet despite his accomplishments, he experienced frequent bouts of intense anxiety and had already developed an ulcer.

Malcolm and I made use of Matrix Nutrition (see Chapter 5) to rework his diet and support his healing. He was also struck by the idea of viewing each moment as a challenge to overcome reactivity and develop his proactive nature (see Chapter 7), particularly since he had already noticed that his ulcer was a reliable—if painful—indicator of his mental and emotional state. The stomach pangs he felt each time he fell prey to worry, anxiety, or insecurity were a powerful reminder of how important it was to find serenity and peace. Yet, of all the tools offered by Matrix Healing, Malcolm was most drawn to the technology embodied in the Names of God, and in kabbalistic techniques for prayer and meditation.

Malcolm had been raised a devout Christian, although he no longer belonged to a church. Despite our vastly different backgrounds, he and I shared a common response to prayer. Both of us had been put off by people we'd known in our childhood and early adulthood who had viewed prayer as a kind of humble supplication, cravenly begging favors from a capricious authority. Yet each of us had had personal experiences with prayer that felt empowering and illuminating. Malcolm admitted that he'd never been sure how to access this sense of empowerment. Sometimes he felt it; other times it eluded him. He was excited by the prospect of tapping into this power whenever he liked, and he was relieved that this might have a healing effect on his ulcer.

I explained to Malcolm that, from my perspective, prayer for a human being is like water for a seed. Just like the seed, we have within us all the potential to achieve great things, but the seed needs water to unlock its potential and, likewise, we need prayer. In my view, prayer is no more about religion than quantum physics is—it's simply a type of technology through which we can be co-creators of reality. As we saw in Chapters 1, 2, and elsewhere, we already have the power to help create reality and to access parallel universes in which we are already perfectly happy, healthy, and fulfilled. Prayer is an enormously effective technology for activating that power, and the Matrix Healing "software" explained at the end of this chapter is a particularly effective use of the technology.

I told Malcolm about the Bible verse in which God responds to the Hebrew people who are trying to escape Egypt and are asking for Him to part the Red Sea. "Why do you cry to me?" God says. On first reading, of course, it's tempting to ask, "Well, who else should they cry to?" But a deeper understanding reveals that God was saying to all of us, "You have the power to be a Co-Creator when you bond with Me. You yourselves can split the Red Sea because you have the power of mind to alter the course of the cosmos, to change the outcome of events." This, I told Malcolm, was how the ancients always understood the world, in which prayer enabled us to form a relationship with universal forces in order to create change.

This, I went on, is why Dr. Larry Dossey is so passionate about the role of prayer in medicine. He sees how powerful this force can be, and so he is always knocking on the door of conventional medicine, trying to wake up physicians to the extraordinary power at their disposal—if they would only use it. Indeed, prayer is, I believe, the most powerful force in creation available to us, a force that can literally change the course of our lives.

"Remember," I told Malcolm, "when you begin to pray, you're entering the Matrix, a dimension that's beyond space, time, and motion, where past, present, and future are merged into one and all possible outcomes are before you. With your own energy, you can direct the course of your life and the future outcomes that will affect you. But only prayer that is deeply rooted in compassion and humility has that kind of power."

Malcolm's religious background had made him open to the concept of prayer. I've had other patients, though, who came from a secular background and who were interested only in a strictly scientific perspective. With them, I focused on the groundbreaking work of psychiatrist and research scientist Jeffrey Schwartz, M.D., whose pioneering work with obsessive-compulsive disorder (OCD) patients is described in the book he wrote with Sharon Begley, *The Mind and the Brain.* (For more on Schwartz's work, see Chapters 2, 5, and 7.)

Obsessive-compulsive disorder is a syndrome in which patients feel compelled to engage in behavior that is seemingly beyond their control—the repetitive washing of hands, for example, or meaningless counting rituals. In *The Mind and the Brain,* Schwartz explains that he was able to help OCD patients overcome their disorder by showing them how to master the faulty brain biochemistry that compelled them to engage in unwanted behavior. OCD patients felt as though their repetitive counting or obsessive rituals were true expressions of their wishes, feelings, and desires, and they experienced enormous despair at being compelled to engage in these meaningless and absurd behaviors. But when they learned that these desires were an illusion, the product of a chemical imbalance rather than of their true selves, they were able to move beyond the unwanted behavior to make healthier—and more pleasant—choices.

Schwartz's patients discovered an enormous sense of liberation when they realized that their true selves were not petty, compulsive, and trapped but, rather, large, empowered, and free. This liberation came from simply saying no to the portion of their brains that insisted on acting compulsively. Both the kabbalistic perspective and Schwartz's scientific point of view come to a similar conclusion: the only power we truly have is the power to resist our egos.

Thus, Schwartz points out that when his patients suffered from OCD symptoms, they were purely passive recipients of their brains' faulty messages. When they undertook his four-step process for overcoming those symptoms, however, they became active and empowered—and this seizing control of their own destinies had a powerful healing effect.

Schwartz goes on to link his scientific discoveries to the Buddhist notion of mindfulness—a detached awareness of each moment that is best practiced through meditation. The only true power we have, he says, lies in the way we respond to our own thoughts: "For Buddhist mindfulness practice, it is the moment of restraint that allows mindful awareness to take hold and deepen . . . to stop the grinding machine-like automaticity of the urge to act. . . . The only willful choice one has is the quality of attention one gives to a thought at any moment." Thus, our power comes from our ability to "just say no" to reactive behavior. Refusing to respond impulsively—or compulsively—gives us access to the godlike power of our true selves.

THE MEDICAL BENEFITS OF PRAYER AND MEDITATION

The town rabbi was unusual in one respect: he had made several business investments in the next town. Yet through an unusual set of misfortunes, every one of these investments failed completely within the same week. The day this unhappy news was learned, the rabbi's disciples were sure that their teacher would be devastated. They rushed to his home to offer comfort and support—only to find him serenely engaged in prayer and study, as he was every morning.

"Rabbi, haven't you heard the news?" asked one disciple. "Your money is all gone—you've lost everything. Aren't you worried?"

The rabbi smiled. "I know this news has brought me many worries," he said calmly. "But God has blessed me with a quick brain. The worrying that other people do in a month, I'm able to finish in an hour or so."

—TRADITIONAL JEWISH FOLKTALE, ADAPTED FROM
A TREASURY OF JEWISH FOLKLORE,
EDITED BY NATHAN AUSUBEL

Later in this chapter, I'll share with you the specific technology of kabbalistic prayer—the Matrix Healing software that can bring you health and anything else you desire. But just to remind you that I am a physician and scientist, let me start by sharing the scientific studies showing the therapeutic effects of meditation, prayer, and other mental self-help techniques. In this materialistic age, it's good to know that medical research confirms what the kabbalists have always known: that prayer, meditation, and your attitude toward the world can have an enormous impact on your health.

Let's begin with the work of Professor David Spiegel, who actually set out not to prove the link between mental attitude and health but, rather, to refute it by showing that the progress of metastatic breast cancer in women was unaffected by their mental states. For ten years, Spiegel followed some eighty-two women with breast cancer, only to discover that his hypothesis was completely wrong. The women who had gotten group therapy and assistance with such techniques as self-hypnosis lived an average of twice as long as those given only the traditional treat-ment. Spiegel himself was stunned by the results, particularly since they were the opposite of what he had intended to prove.

Likewise, Carl and Stephanie Simonton demonstrated a dou-bling of survival rates in cancer patients who used imagery and visualization to slow the spread of cancer cells and overcome the disease. Although visualization, imagery, and self-hypnosis are not identical with prayer, they call upon the same powerful resource: the Light within our own souls, with which we have the ability to heal ourselves anytime we choose.

Researchers who have specifically studied prayer have agreed that it can be a remarkably effective healing tool. According to Jeff Levin, M.D., author of *God, Faith, and Health: Exploring the Spirituality-Healing Connection,* prayer was associated with better health among every type of religious and ethnic group. One study Levin reports concerned more than 500 Mexican Ameri-cans and Anglo Caucasians. The longer and more frequently members of each group prayed, the greater well-being they enjoyed more than eight years later. Another study revealed similar results for African Americans.

According to Levin and his fellow researchers, the benefit of prayer or religious devotion was not due to social reasons—the help of fellow church members, for example, or the good repu-tation one acquires as a "person of faith." Rather, the health ben-efits came from the way that the prayerful or religious person could tap into a sense of optimism and joy—what Matrix Heal-ers would call certainty. (For more on certainty, see Chapter 2.) Both their physical condition and their mental state improved from this access to another dimension—the dimension I think of as the Matrix.

Likewise, in another study, of 4,000 adults in North Carolina, researchers examined the effects of religious devotion by asking subjects about such activities as prayer, meditation, and Bible study. They also asked people to rate their own health. According to the study, the more frequently people participated in prayer, meditation, and the exploration of religious texts, the more likely they were to report themselves as healthy, regardless of the actual state of their health. This self-rating is known as "subjective health," and it's considered a significant indicator of a person's overall state of health, as well as one of the best predictors of longevity.

A study entitled "Meditation Reduces Medical Costs" provides further support for the notion that prayer, meditation, and related activities are good for our health. This preliminary study, conducted in Quebec, Canada, focused on Transcendental Meditation (TM), a type of meditation that involves 15- to 20-minute sessions of focused yet relaxed concentration. Researchers analyzed the payments made to physicians by some 677 people who had begun practicing TM. For the three years before their involvement with TM, the subjects' doctor bills remained unchanged. As soon as the subjects began engaging in TM, however, their doctor bills went down 5 to 7 percent each year.

This study had no control group—no comparable group of people who did *not* practice TM. Perhaps many others in Quebec saw a general decline in medical bills, or perhaps there was some other reason for this group's apparently improved health. Moreover, the people in the study had all chosen to study TM, making them a rather unusual segment of the population, perhaps one that was already healthier or more prone to health improvements than other people. Nevertheless, because the study involved so many people and produced such dramatic results, it remains an impressive suggestion that meditation is good for your health.

So far, we've considered the effect of prayer and meditation on the health of the person who meditates or prays. But what effect do our prayers have on other people? In one famous study conducted by the San Francisco cardiologist Randolph C. Byrd and published in 1988 in the *Southern Medical Journal*, 393 patients in a cardiac care unit were randomly divided into two groups. One set of patients was prayed for by Christian prayer groups from a distant location, while the other set of patients was simply treated as usual. In this double-blind study, neither the patients, the people who cared for them, nor the researchers knew who was in which group. The people who prayed never met or even saw the people they prayed for. They were simply given the patients' names, diagnoses, and general condition. They were not told where the patients were located or given any other identifying information.

The results were astonishing. Patients who were prayed for had fewer cases of congestive heart failure, cardiac arrest, and pneumonia. They were discharged earlier, intubated less often, and generally needed fewer medications and lower dosages.

Dr. Elisabeth Targ and her colleagues at California Pacific Medical Center in San Francisco conducted a similar study of distant healing with prayer, this time on forty patients with advanced cases of AIDS. Twenty of these patients received distant healing prayer along with their regular care, while twenty received only regular care. None of the patients was aware of which group he or she was in. Each person who prayed was given only a first name and a photograph of the patient he or she was to pray for.

The people praying focused their consciousness on the patient's health and well-being for one hour a day, six days a week, for ten weeks. The patients were evaluated after six months. The group who had received the prayer treatments had significantly fewer new AIDS-related illnesses and fewer doctor visits and hospitalizations. In addition, their moods were significantly better.

Clearly, in both the Byrd and the Targ studies, some connective energy had passed from those who prayed to those who were prayed for—not unlike the energy flowing from the drunkard to the rabbi in the story that opened this chapter.

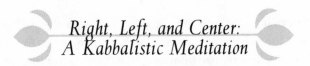

Right, Left, and Center: A Kabbalistic Meditation

PREPARATION

Use the same deep-breathing preparation recommended for "Balancing *Chochma* and *Bina*" in Chapter 3. Conscious breathing is a great way to tap into our own power, as we mirror the Creator's original act of breathing life into the universe.

MEDITATION

This exercise is adapted from a meditation developed by Mark Cohen, Ph.D.

1. Allow your attention to focus on the right side of your body, what the kabbalists call the right column. Recall that this column represents the Desire to Give. It is the part of our energy that is already exactly like that of the Creator. Within the domain of this energy, we are God-like, powerful, creative, and proactive. We are beings of total compassion, love, and sharing. We are whole and complete, already healed, already perfect, just as God is perfect. Enter deeply into this side of your being. Experience your wholeness, your power, your compassion. Remain within the right column for 5 minutes.

2. Now bring your attention to the left side of your body, the so-called left column. This column represents the Desire to Receive.

It is the portion of us that has not yet attained unity with the Creator, the place where we are limited, reactive, frustrated, ill. Experience this part of your being as fully as you can. Allow yourself to feel how much you desire to receive the healing Light and love of the Creator, how incomplete and vulnerable you are. Remain within the left column for 5 minutes.

3. Return to the right column for another 5 minutes, then to the left column for an equal amount of time. You can move on to step 4, or continue to alternate from right to left for up to a total of 30 minutes on each side. (More than 30 minutes total on the left side is not recommended, as it gives too much power to this aspect of your being.)

4. Finally, hold both sides in your mind at the same time. Feel a new dimension emerge—the central column—integrating both the right and the left sides of your being. Allow this new dimension to spread slowly through your heart, mind, and spirit, throughout your entire body, and into your soul. Spend at least 5 minutes immersed in central-column energy before you end the meditation and return to your daily life.

 Facing the Fears That Hold You Back

PREPARATION

Use the same deep-breathing preparation recommended for "Balancing *Chochma* and *Bina*" in Chapter 3. Remember that conscious breathing is an excellent aid in any effort to overcome reactive behavior, since in breathing, we are partaking of the Creator's original act of breathing life into the universe. Our breath also cools the hot, reactive behavior of the heart and liver.

EXERCISE

This exercise is adapted from *The Magic Book,* prepared by the Kabbalah Centre.

1. As your mind clears with the preparation described above, allow yourself to focus on a particular intention. Formulate this intention so that it becomes as specific as possible. Don't just say, "I'd like a better relationship with my husband," but rather, "Help me be able to give and receive more love with my husband," or "I'd like to spend more time laughing and just enjoying life with my husband." Knowing exactly what you want is part of tapping into the power of getting it.

2. Write down your intention, keeping the words as specific as possible. You may find that this process of formulating and writing is itself one of exploration. Perhaps you'll begin with one notion in mind and realize that you don't actually want it after all, but something very different. Or maybe you'll affirm your original desires but get in touch with exactly what you mean by such general phrases as "I wish I had a girlfriend," or "I'd like to be more successful." At any rate, continue with the process until you have written down a clear, specific intention that feels right to you.

3. Now shut your eyes and visualize getting exactly what you've asked for. What fears, anxieties, and concerns come up? You can be sure that *some* kind of block will arise at this point; otherwise, you would already have the thing you desire or be well on your way to getting it. Without judgment or self-blame, allow your concerns to enter your consciousness, however irrational, selfish, or problematic they might seem.

4. Open your eyes and write down a list of each fear or worry you have about achieving your goal. For example, if your goal is success at work, you may find yourself thinking, "All my co-workers will be mad at me—they'll think I'm arrogant and power-hungry." If your

goal is a better relationship with your spouse, you may think, "I'll become too dependent on my marriage and stop being my own person." Allow yourself to be as clear, specific, and honest as possible about what's in your way.

5. Write down your list of fears, concerns, and blocks. You might want to copy your thoughts onto a clean sheet of paper, so you can clearly see your intention and your list of fears.

6. Close your eyes and tap into the power of the Light. Feel the Light entering your body and spirit through *Keter*, the *Sefira* at the crown of your head. Feel it filtering down through *Chochma, Bina, Da'at, Chesed, Gevurah, Tiferet, Netzach, Hod, Yesod,* and *Malchut*—from right to left to central column. (If necessary, review Chapter 3 before beginning this exercise.) Take a moment to experience the sensation of each *Sefira* as it glows with warm, loving Light. See each *Sefira's* unique color and feel the special quality of its energy. Visualize your body and spirit illuminated at each *Sefira,* alive with the Creator's Light—*your* Light.

7. Again, open your eyes. Look at each fear you have listed and write what you see as a spiritual and practical response to each one. For example, if your concern is that financial success is going to make you a selfish or greedy person, your spiritual response might be to remember that you have the power to become exactly the kind of person you want to be, no matter what your circumstances. Your practical response might be to pledge a certain percentage of your income to charity now, with a commitment to enlarging that pledge as you become more successful.

8. When you have finished the process of writing solutions, close your eyes and reconnect to the Light in each *Sefira.* Breathe deeply for a few moments, experiencing the expansion of Light that you have just allowed into your own personal Tree of Life.

THE HEALING POWER OF EMPATHY

> A rabbi was known for his strict observance of Jewish law. Typically, in the weeks before Passover, he himself supervised the preparation of the matzohs, so he could guarantee that every single religious regulation was observed.
>
> One year, though, the rabbi fell ill and his disciples offered to supervise the matzoh-baking in his place. "Just tell us what to watch out for," they asked their teacher.
>
> "There's only one thing that really matters," the rabbi replied. "Make sure the women who bake the matzohs are well paid."
>
> —JEWISH FOLKTALE, ADAPTED FROM *A TREASURY OF JEWISH FOLKLORE*, EDITED BY NATHAN AUSUBEL

If I were to leave you with only one thought about using prayer in Matrix Healing, it would be this: only when we experience true compassion can we become truly healed.

The rabbi in the folktale understood that all the protocols of piety, all the regulations and laws set down by any religion—Judaism, Christianity, Islam, Buddhism—mean very little beside the overriding power of compassion. Without this compassion, we can never truly heal others. We cannot even heal ourselves.

People tend to misunderstand the notion of compassion, based on centuries of materialistic thinking. Remember the mechanistic worldview developed by Isaac Newton and others, in which subjective responses were seen as completely separate from objective reality? (See Chapter 1.) This split between ourselves and the outer world was mirrored in the thinking of eighteenth-century French philosopher René Descartes. Descartes claimed that the entire world existed in four dimensions: the three physical dimensions of location, breadth, and height, and the fourth dimension of time. In this way of thinking, bodies were separated from one another by space and time. I am one person, standing here; you are a separate person, standing over there. I am one person, existing now; you are someone else entirely, existing four hundred years ago or four hundred years in the future. In this view, the world is a collection of unrelated objects and people, with no intrinsic connection to one another.

Thus, in this Cartesian worldview, I have no real need to feel compassion for you. At best, feeling compassion or empathy is optional—a praiseworthy act, to be sure, but one that has no real relationship to my own inner nature, let alone to my physical health. If you and I are separate beings, all I really have to do is take care of myself—*my* body, *my* mental state, *my* spiritual balance sheet. You are basically irrelevant to my identity, and you are certainly irrelevant to my health.

That's very different from how the kabbalists view the world. Kabbalah is based on the notion that everything in the world is intrinsically connected. The tiniest part contains the whole, while the whole reflects the condition of every one of its parts. Past, present, and future are all one, so that when we pour poison into the oceans, for example, we are wounded along with the future generations who are left to clean up our mess. Likewise, we ourselves were freed from Egypt along with the Hebrews; we ourselves overcame segregation with the civil rights movement; we ourselves suffered with the victims of the Holocaust and the slave trade, even if we have the illusion of having been born only a few years ago.

In the kabbalistic view, it is as ridiculous for me to view myself as separate from you as it would be for our kidneys to view themselves as separate from our hearts. If the heart is sick, the kidneys are affected. Although on one level, it makes sense to consider them as two distinct entities, on another level, seeing them as separate is absurd.

Likewise, if you injure yourself as a child, you carry the scars into adulthood. There's no meaning in separating your four-year-old bout with polio or asthma from the adult condition of your legs or lungs—it's all one body, with one living history.

In the same way, according to Kabbalah, we are all part of one another, of all creation and all history. If we believe that our health can be separated from the health of our fellow humans or from the health of our planet, we are as deluded as if we believed that a heart attack or an infected finger affects only one small part of the body. Only when we view the human race and our entire world as a single, interrelated whole can we find true health.

We'll talk more about this ecological view in Chapter 9. For now, it's important to remember that having this larger vision is a crucial part of employing the kabbalistic technology of prayer. Only when we feel compassion for others as well as ourselves— only when we see that what affects our world affects us—can we tap into the true power of the Matrix.

THE BUILDING BLOCKS OF CREATION

> [T] he supernal letters . . . brought into being all the works of the lower world, literally after their own pattern.
>
> —THE ZOHAR

One of the aspects of Matrix prayer that Malcolm found most fascinating was the role of the Hebrew letters. According to Kabbalah, these letters have a very different status from any other alphabet. They are the very building blocks of creation, the embodiment of the energy that brought forth our world. Indeed, the Hebrew word for "letter" really means "pulse" or "vibration."

It's a mistake to think of the Hebrew alphabet the way we think of any other, or to think of the Names of God as actual names. They're almost like scientific symbols—H_2O, for example, or $E = MC^2$—except that the letters do not merely represent energy. They actually *are* energy. And when you scan or meditate upon each of these names, you access the same creative forces that brought our world into being.

When I first told Malcolm about the remarkable power of the Hebrew alphabet, he felt both skeptical and intimidated. "It's a little hard for me to accept that any one people has a monopoly on sacred energy," he said frankly. "And besides, I don't know Hebrew. So what use are these names to me?"

I explained to Malcolm that these particular letters and their sequences are *not* confined to one people. Rather, they are universal symbols that transcend religion, race, geography, and the very concept of language as we know it. They were intended for all people to use to interact with our universe and, ultimately, to control their own destinies.

As a result, I told Malcolm, it's not important whether you understand Hebrew or not. All you have to do is scan the letters, open your mind to their hidden power, and allow them to unlock your own creative energies. The rest is up to you.

MIND OVER MATTER: A FOUR-STEP PROGRAM

A wonder-working rabbi had died, and his bereft disciples went to the widow, each hoping to purchase one of the great man's possessions as a kind of keepsake. One of the disciples caught sight of the rabbi's pipe—a lovely wooden object with an elaborately painted porcelain bowl. The rabbi's wife was asking a high price for the pipe, so the disciple asked permission to take it home and try it out. Sitting in front of his fireside, the disciple lit the rabbi's pipe and began to smoke. To his amazement, he was immediately seized with an extraordinary vision of the Other World. He saw angels, archangels, and all sorts of heavenly spirits. Transfixed, he continued to puff until finally the vision evaporated.

The disciple hurried back to the rabbi's wife, paid her the price she'd asked, and went home again to relight the miraculous pipe. This time, however, nothing out of the ordinary happened.

Devastated by disappointment, the disciple went to the new rabbi to ask for an explanation. The new rabbi listened carefully to his story. Then he smiled. "The first time you smoked the pipe, it still belonged to the rabbi," he explained. "So when you smoked it, you saw what the rabbi saw. But the second time you smoked it, it belonged to you. So you saw only what *you* see."

–TRADITIONAL JEWISH FOLKTALE, ADAPTED FROM
A TREASURY OF JEWISH FOLKLORE,
EDITED BY NATHAN AUSUBEL

As the story of the rabbi's pipe makes clear, it's not enough simply to believe in other universes or other states of being. We have to know *how* to access them. Fortunately, Kabbalah gives us the software that truly enables us to make "mind over matter" a reality. But we have to do our part. The Names of God are not here to magically grant us wishes while we remain idle and unchanged. Rather, they are here to help us with the difficult but exhilarating work of personal transformation. From being a person who is laid low by disease, we suddenly become a person who is healthy. From being a person who has no loving partner, we suddenly become a person who is capable of having one. Or rather, in both cases, we access that portion of ourselves that is already healthy, already beloved—we access that God-like portion of ourselves that is creative, proactive, loving, and free. Like Schwartz's OCD patients, we say *no* to the portion of our brain that insists we are sick, lonely, or confined to a role we no longer want. The prayer accesses our power—but to truly make use of our power, we still have to take action.

Here, then, is a four-step process for using the Names of God and other Hebrew prayers. As you'll see, it involves both sharing and receiving, both accessing the Creator's power and tapping into our own. Learning to pray in this way may take some time. Stick with it, though—the results may be beyond anything you've ever imagined.

Step 1: Know the Laws of the Universe

I hope you've already completed Step 1 through the process of reading this book. You understand the concepts of Light and the Vessel, the notion of synthesizing the Desire to Share and the Desire to Receive into a new desire—the Desire to Receive for the Sake of Sharing. You have mastered the concept of the Matrix—that alternate universe in which everything is possible and you have infinite access to the Creator's power. Whether you call that reality God, the Creator, the Light, the Life Force, or any other name you choose, you understand that it is a loving, creative, proactive force that we can all tap into. You're ready to overcome Bread of Shame by sharing your true essence with your fellow humans, your planet, and the universe at large. And you know that the most important thing in life is overcoming your reactive nature, becoming the proactive, creative, loving person that, in the Matrix, you already are. In the words of the great kabbalist Rav Cook, "Every person needs to know that he is called to serve based on the model of perception and feeling which is unique to him, based on the core root of his soul. In that root, which contains infinite worlds, he will find the treasure of his life. A person needs to say, *'Bishvili nivrah ha-olam'* [The world was created for me]."

Step 2: Be in a State of Empathy and Compassion

To achieve this state, you've got to significantly diminish ego, not just to be "a better person" but because ego will block your prayer. Becoming wholly absorbed in empathy and compassion, on the other hand, enables you to open up the channels of prayer. Empathy is not some nice thing you do for extra credit. It's a recognition of the most profound reality of your existence, an understanding of how your identity and destiny are inextricably bound with the entire universe, just as the identity and destiny of your heart is inextricably bound with your entire body. In this state of humility and compassion, we are in this wholeness.

This integrated reality is the Matrix, that parallel universe that quantum physics tells us is floating out there and which Kabbalah tells us how to access. Both our universe and the Matrix change in response to real changes. And when you truly understand that mind and matter are one—because we are all one with the Creator—you will be able to heal yourself. But the only way to grasp this truth is to feel compassion and empathy, because these emotions remind you that there is no real distinction between yourself and any other aspect of our universe. When you have grasped that ultimate meaning, you will be able to heal—or to accomplish any other task you choose.

Step 3. Become Absorbed in the Experience You Wish to Achieve

In other words, if you want to be healed, then feel, emote, and think as though you were already healed. If you want to find a life partner, become the person who is already deeply and satisfyingly beloved. If you want to achieve more success at work, experience all the emotions you know will accompany that achievement, and think the way you will think when you have reached that goal. Do it *now*—in other words, close the gap between yourself and your desires by becoming the person *now* that you wish to be *then*.

This is not simply an empty exercise in "the power of positive thinking." You may have noticed that often, when you meet a stranger, you can tell instantly whether that person has a happy love life or an enjoyable job. Something in his or her actions, energy, and demeanor communicates a powerful message. Or perhaps you have friends you admire in one domain or another. When you run into difficulties, you find yourself thinking, "This sort of thing doesn't happen to so-and-so—I can't imagine her putting up with it," or "I can't imagine him letting this stop him." The people who have achieved the goals you seek got there by acting, feeling, and thinking in a particular way. When you assume that way of being, you'll achieve the same goals. So as you pray, allow yourself to experience that desired state with the certainty that you, too, will achieve your heart's desire.

Step 4. Make Use of the Hebrew Letters

Hebrew letters and sequences help bridge the gap between mind and matter. So once you have understood the laws of the universe, felt compassion and humility, and reached forward to the state you desire, you may want to access the power that comes from Hebrew letters, scanning some of the sequences and prayers shown below. After you have used deep, conscious breathing to put yourself into a receptive state (you might use the preparation exercise from Chapter 3), simply scan these letters, from right to left, again and again, for a period lasting 5 to 15 minutes.

You can also use just one of the seventy-two names, the *Mem Hay Shin*. Prepare yourself with conscious breathing and then scan the letters again and again for 5 to 15 minutes as you allow their healing energy to penetrate your body, mind, and spirit. You might also repeat this sequence of letters phonetically, aloud or in your mind.

מהש׳

Another powerful healing tool is the *Ana-bakoach* (a-na-ba-KO-akh), a sequence of forty-two letters decoded by the kabbalists from the beginning of the Torah, which describes the creation process. The *Ana-bakoach* includes seven lines, which you can scan one at a time, again from right to left. The first line is a code that helps us tap into the energy of unconditional love. The second line enables us to remove any negative thoughts, lingering doubts, or reactive consciousness that continues to impede our progress. The third line is to help us start anew. It evokes the energy of sustenance and healing, particularly that aspect of healing that involves returning to the beginning and starting over.

For healing, the first three lines of the *Ana-bakoach* are the most important, but all seven lines work together. So again, prepare yourself with a breathing exercise and then give yourself 5 to 15 minutes to scan these letters, line by line. As you scan the first three lines, you might allow the concepts I've described to float into your mind, but as you proceed to the last four lines, allow your mind to become clear. Just let the visual image of the letters work upon you at your deepest level.

אָנָּא בְּכֹחַ, גְּדֻלַּת יְמִינְךָ, תַּתִּיר צְרוּרָה:
קַבֵּל רִנַּת, עַמְּךָ שַׂגְּבֵנוּ, טַהֲרֵנוּ נוֹרָא:
נָא גִּבּוֹר, דּוֹרְשֵׁי יִחוּדְךָ, כְּבָבַת שָׁמְרֵם:
בָּרְכֵם טַהֲרֵם, רַחֲמֵי צִדְקָתֶךָ, תָּמִיד גָּמְלֵם:
חֲסִין קָדוֹשׁ, בְּרוֹב טוּבְךָ, נַהֵל עֲדָתֶךָ:
יָחִיד גֵּאֶה, לְעַמְּךָ פְּנֵה, זוֹכְרֵי קְדֻשָּׁתֶךָ:
שַׁוְעָתֵנוּ קַבֵּל, וּשְׁמַע צַעֲקָתֵנוּ, יוֹדֵעַ תַּעֲלוּמוֹת:
אָנָּא בְּכֹחַ, גְּדֻלַּת יְמִינְךָ, תַּתִּיר צְרוּר
קַבֵּל רִנַּת, עַמְּךָ שַׂגְּבֵנוּ, טַהֲרֵנוּ נוֹרָא:
נָא גִּבּוֹר, דּוֹרְשֵׁי יִחוּדְךָ, כְּבָבַת שָׁמְרֵם:

There is also the healing sequence devised by Moses to heal his sister Miriam, the prophetess. Again, clear your mind, breathe deeply, and scan the letters. You can also repeat them phonetically in your mind again and again, or repeat them softly aloud.

אֵל נָא רְפָא נָא לָהּ

Finally, you can use the *Raphaynu*, which I often prescribe to my patients. The words of this prayer literally mean, "God heal us—and we are healed!" As you can see, the first portion of the prayer is the voicing of our intention to be healed, while the second portion is the affirmation that we *are* healed as soon as we express the intent.

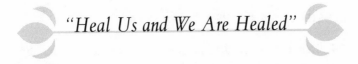

"Heal Us and We Are Healed"

PREPARATION

Use the same deep-breathing preparation recommended for "Balancing *Chochma* and *Bina*" in Chapter 3.

MEDITATION

1. Breathe in and out, focusing on the breath. Remember that each breath links you with the breath of the cosmos, for the Light breathed into humanity is the breath of life. Feel your own life force growing stronger with every breath.

2. As you breathe, visualize the state of health you wish to occupy. Experience the state of health that you desire.

3. Affirm your certainty that this perfect health is the true basis of the world. Know that everything is whole, flowing, connected, healed. Feel this perfection. Visualize it. See yourself already healed in your mind's eye.

4. Say aloud "Raphaynu Yud-Hay-Vov-Hay V'nai Rafei/Heal us, O God, and we are healed."

ACCESSING THE POWER OF PRAYER

> A disciple once asked his rabbi what the rabbi did before he prayed.
>
> The rabbi replied, "I pray that when I pray, it should be with my whole heart."
>
> —TRADITIONAL JEWISH FOLKTALE, ADAPTED FROM
> *A TREASURY OF JEWISH FOLKLORE,*
> EDITED BY NATHAN AUSUBEL

As I was in the midst of writing this chapter, I had my own profound experience with the power of prayer. My brother's wife gave birth to her daughter prematurely—after only twenty-six weeks of pregnancy. The infant weighed less than two pounds at the time I flew down to see her. I admit that although—or perhaps because—I was a physician, I felt a certain trepidation about seeing this tiny child, knowing how sick she would be and what an uncertain prognosis most doctors would give her.

Yet the moment I saw her, I felt overcome by such a powerful wave of compassion, I was almost unable to speak—a compassion that soon transformed itself into an equally powerful joy. Despite all the problems my niece was facing, I realized that it was an extraordinary experience to feel the love and Light she brought with her into the world.

As I stood near her crib, I began saying the letters of one of the seventy-two names to myself, repeating *Mem Hay Shin* again and again in my mind. Suddenly, with an energy she had not shown before, the infant opened her eyes and stared at me. I felt a calm certainty that we were sharing the language of the soul. Although on one level, *Mem Hay Shin* is merely a meaningless sequence of letters, on another level, my niece and I were communicating, soul to soul, and I could see that this connection was having a powerful healing effect on both of us.

I began to say the *El nah Repha na lah*, the sequence of letters that Moses discovered in order to save his sister Miriam. It seemed to me that my niece responded with even more intensity, creating a soul bond between us so great that we both resonated with it profoundly, as though this were a language that she had known through eternity, a language that I, too, had once known, forgotten, and had finally rediscovered.

My niece has been recovering slowly but steadily since that visit, and each time I see her, I spend several minutes reconnecting on this soul level. Although I had shared with many patients the following words of St. Francis of Assisi, I have now finally begun to understand them for myself:

> Lord, make me an instrument of your peace:
> Where there is hatred, let me sow love.
> Where there is injury, pardon.
> Where there is discord, union.
> Where there is doubt, faith.
> Where there is despair, hope.
> Where there is darkness, light.
> And where there is sadness, joy.
> Divine Master, grant that I may not so much seek to be
> consoled, as to console;
> to be understood, as to understand;
> to be loved, as to love;
> for it is in giving that we receive.
> It is in pardoning that we are pardoned.
> And it is in dying that we are born to eternal life.

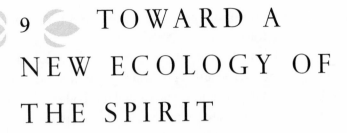

9 TOWARD A NEW ECOLOGY OF THE SPIRIT

> *I will give you a new heart, and a new spirit, and a new heaven, and a new earth.*

MY patient Rosa was an intense, ambitious woman in her early thirties who had come to me with an underfunctioning thyroid. The list of symptoms associated with hypothyroidism is long and distressing, and Rosa had suffered from most of them, including fatigue, weight gain, constipation, hair loss, "brain fog," excessive menstrual flow, and muscle aches. She'd called me after I'd helped a friend of hers who'd been struggling with chronic fatigue syndrome, which can be one result of low thyroid function. Rosa was struck by how many of her symptoms resembled those of her friend, even though she hadn't received the same diagnosis.

I treated Rosa with the usual supplements and dietary suggestions, which are key to treating hypothyroidism, especially in women. Rosa had always been a psychologically-minded person, so she was also open to the idea that the disease she carried represented an aspect of her personality and a spiritual lesson that she needed to learn.

Actually, I thought Rosa was almost too receptive to the idea that her illness was the direct physical expression of her personal psychology. While I certainly believe that our bodies tell our stories, I am not comfortable with the idea that each illness simply represents an individual's problem. I've come to see illness as something larger than just one person, something that tells the story of our society—indeed, of our humanity.

In Rosa's case, for example, her hypothyroidism had many causes, but at least some of them were environmental. Radiation interferes with thyroid function, and Rosa lived in New York City, where she worked as a secretary. So she was continually exposed to the radiation from the computers and electronic equipment at her job, while every time she left the house she was bombarded by the radiation from power stations, microwaves, cell phones, and other kinds of machinery—not to mention the residual nuclear radiation from accidents such as the one at Chernobyl.

At least in part, then, Rosa's disease told the story not just of her own body but also of the environment in which she lived—an environment full of radiation, machines, and other threats to human health. Perhaps her disease also told the story of her spiritual environment. Couldn't we see both Rosa's hypothyroidism and her friend's chronic fatigue syndrome as resulting from a kind of spiritual fatigue, representing the exhaustion and depression of our entire society?

So as I treated Rosa for her specific symptoms, I also shared with her my sense of spiritual ecology. In the past thirty years, we've come to accept the principles of natural ecology—the notion that all life systems on earth are literally connected. Smokestacks in Michigan can create acid rain in the South

Pacific. A nuclear accident in Chernobyl can poison milk in the United Kingdom. I've even read recently that the increased carbon dioxide in our atmosphere, discharged by automobiles and factories of all types, may actually be changing the patterns of how the earth revolves.

In exactly the same way, I told Rosa, Kabbalah teaches that we are connected to all other humans on earth, physically and spiritually. As long as any one of us has a disease, we all have that disease. If any one of us is unenlightened, none of us is completely enlightened. Certainly it's important to take individual responsibility for our spiritual and physical health. But we are not *only* individuals. Just as Rosa was affected by the radiation surrounding her, so was she affected by the physical and spiritual condition of the people in her world. If there is violence or disorder anywhere in the world, I told her, then there will be disorder within the workings of every person's immune system.

Rosa was happy to embrace the concept of spiritual ecology. She readily agreed that her health was affected by factors that went beyond her individual life, and she was inspired by the idea that we "carry" each other's diseases, just as we benefit from each other's health. "I'll do what I can to get better" is the way she put it, "and I like knowing that the Matrix is there for me to 'plug into.' But I also like knowing that I'm part of something larger—that my disease is not just *my* disease, but part of the whole world I live in. Of course, I want to get better. But I want my world to get better, too."

Rosa's words reminded me of the ancient Jewish concept of *tikkun olam*—to mend, repair, and transform the world. Kabbalah teaches that together we can create a world of abundance, joy, and prosperity—a world of health and well-being for everyone. That, I believe, is the true meaning of Kabbalah.

THE ART OF CONNECTION

> Only connect.
>
> —E. M. FORSTER, *HOWARDS END*

As we've seen in previous chapters, Matrix Healing is all about the art of connection—restoring our profound, healing connection to ourselves and each other as well as to nature, our planet, and, ultimately, to the Light, the mystery, the source of sources, so that all of creation forms one unified whole. In the words of the Zohar:

> *I have seen that all those sparks flash from the High Spark.* . . .
> *All those lights are connected:*
> *this light to that light, that light to this light,*
> *one shining into the other,*
> *inseparable one from the other.*

Or, to quote Abraham Abulafia, the great kabbalist of the early Middle Ages, "Now we are no longer separated from our source, and behold we are the source and the source is us. We are so intimately united with It we cannot by any means be separated from It, for we are It."

From various perspectives, we've seen how important this spirit of connection can be to our physical, psychological, and spiritual health. To offer only one tiny example of how connectedness can be good for our health, studies have shown that patients in burn units do better in shared rooms than in private ones. Apparently, knowing that they are not alone, and having the chance to cheer each other on, is enormously helpful to burn patients—as it is to all of us.

If we truly understand the scientific principles of the world in which we live, we begin to see that there is a very good reason wholeness and connection are healthy. It's not simply that they "feel good"—although, of course, they do. It's also that our bodies, minds, and spirits are programmed that way. Just as our bodies work better when we eat clean, pure foods and breathe fresh air, so do our souls and spirits work better when we are part of a larger whole.

The human need for connection is clearly recognized by the Torah, which, in all its pages, names only one thing as "not good"—humans being alone. From a Christian perspective, the poet John Milton made the same observation: "The first thing which God's eye nam'd not good was Man being alone."

Larry Dossey is a physician who has written numerous books on the spiritual aspects of healing. His work has meant a great deal to me ever since I first encountered it as a new doctor and felt that here was finally someone in the medical profession with whom I could connect. In *Meaning and Medicine: Lessons from a Doctor's Tales of Breakthrough and Healing,* he describes the work of Dr. Renee Weber, philosopher and professor at Rutgers University, as it applies to this notion of connection and wholeness: "In her seminal paper 'Philosophical Foundations and Frameworks for Healing,' she has proposed that there is an implicit ordering principle at the foundation of existence—a certain wholeness and perfection that surfaces under propitious conditions. The role of the healer is to facilitate this process—to call forth the right order from the void."

Weber further explores this notion of the world's wholeness through a number of philosophical and religious traditions, including the Sankhya philosophy of ancient India, yoga, and Buddhism, as well as via the Greek philosophers Plato and Pythagoras and the Jewish freethinker Spinoza. "Seen against the backdrop of these historical traditions," Dossey writes, "our notion of the void as nothingness and death may seem like a historical aberration."

In other words, the world of chaos, pain, suffering, and misery is, as both Kabbalah and Buddhism would have it, the world of illusion, the static interpretation of a far more dynamic underlying reality—the Matrix. Only ego prevents us from penetrating the mundane deceptions of our everyday lives and perceiving the "really real": that we have the power at any moment to access the Matrix and Tree of Life consciousness, creating for ourselves perfect health, healing, and joy.

On some level, I believe, we're all conscious of this whole and perfect world, even if we also suffer from a kind of ego-generated collective amnesia that blots it out. Certainly, it was the loneliness of not connecting that led us to imagine the bleak and soulless worldview of the mechanistic universe, which viewed the human body as a machine and the human heart as a pump. When we projected our own loneliness onto nature, we created the cold, mechanical world in which we live. Today we are still paying—as doctors, patients, and citizens of the world—for the horrifying limits of that view.

Yet with just a tiny shift in psychological orientation, how beautiful the world becomes! Suddenly even the plants and trees become our companions, and the very hills and mountains take on a life of their own. Think of the animated world King David saw when he wrote, "And the mountains skipped like rams, and the hills like little lambs, and the rivers clapped, and the hills sang." It was this notion of a world full of life that led the sixteenth-century Rabbi Isaac Luria, one of the world's great kabbalists, to write that creation's ultimate purpose is unification, to see the divinity in everything, and to remove all the obstacles that have kept the souls on earth from uniting with one another and with the Light. Such a vision was achieved by one of the few humans to truly get perspective on our planet, an astronaut who described this moment of seeing earth from space: "Instead of an intellectual search, there was suddenly a very deep gut feeling. Knowing for sure that there was a purposefulness of flow, of energy, of time, of space in the cosmos—that it was beyond man's rational ability to understand . . . I suddenly experienced the universe as intelligent, loving, harmonious."

That is our true birthright, which we can access anytime we choose, simply by reaching out.

THE PROBLEM OF EVIL

> Nothing human is alien to me.
>
> —TERENCE, ROMAN POET

Although my patient Rosa was powerfully attracted by the notion of a larger world in which she shared the destiny of every other human being, she balked when it came to thinking about people she considered truly evil. "What about mass murderers?" she asked me. "Or rapists, or Nazis, or any of the other people whose lives are full of hate? How am I supposed to connect to them?"

Of course, philosophers through the ages have wrestled with the problem of evil, and I'm certainly not going to resolve it here! But I did tell Rosa the following story about one of my favorite kabbalists, Israel ben Eliezer, better known as the Baal Shem Tov, or "Master of the Good Name." This rabbi was known as a brilliant scholar who also had a deep love of nature and a profound connection to all living things, and I think this famous tale perfectly captures his deep kindness and his overwhelming love:

When the Baal Shem Tov was only a ten-year-old boy named Israel, he became an orphan, and was raised by the people of his village. He spent most of his time outdoors, absorbing the lessons of nature. He also helped the local schoolmaster care for the younger children, guiding them back and forth between their homes and the schoolhouse. He took the children through the forest, singing beautiful melodies with them, and when the children's joyous music reached Heaven, a rumor began that the time of the Messiah had finally arrived.

Satan heard the rumor and, enraged, asked God to let him challenge these happy children. God agreed, and Satan began his search for someone on earth who would do his work. Since Satan cannot act on his own, but only through the actions of living creatures, he needed an evil messenger.

Not even the smallest ant or the meanest animal would do Satan's bidding to harm the Baal Shem Tov. Finally, he found an old man who had actually been born without a soul and who lived on the edge of the village, avoiding all human contact. Working through this pitiful creature, Satan caused the man to become a werewolf. Then he literally removed the creature's heart and replaced it with his own heart of evil, a dark void within a void.

When Israel and the children confronted this creature emerging from the forest, the children were terrified. But Israel moved forward, even though the evil creature was growing bigger and bigger. Soon, the werewolf's body seemed as enormous as a dark cloud, and Israel found himself literally within the belly of the beast. He was frightened, but he knew the power of certainty, and he knew that wherever he was, there the Light was, too.

Through the foul-smelling shadows of the creature's body, Israel saw the void that was its evil heart. He reached up and took the heart within his own hand. Stepping back, he left the creature's body, still in possession of its heart. Imagine! At that moment,

*Israel held the very heart of evil in his hand. Had he destroyed it,
evil would have vanished from the world.*

*But Israel saw a drop of blood trickling from the heart, and he
felt compassion in his soul. This heart was in agony because it, too,
was suffering the horrible pangs of loneliness that we all feel when
we are separated from the Divine. After all, everything in the
universe is ultimately created by the Light—and all of us, no
matter how evil, feel the tremendous pain that comes with
separation.*

*Moved by compassion, Israel put the heart on the ground, and
the earth instantly swallowed it up. The next day, the villagers
found the body of the werewolf, become a man once more, dead and
still, but with a peaceful look on his face for the first time in his
life. Israel's action reminds us all that nothing on earth, even the
ultimate evil, does not on some level yearn to be returned to its
Divine source. And as long as any of us is separated from the
Light, all of us must suffer.*

OUR POWER TO HEAL

Is it not to share your bread with the hungry

and to take the wretched poor into your home—

when you see the naked, to clothe him,

and not to turn away from your own kin?

Then your light will break forth like the dawn,

and your healing will spring up quickly....

—ISAIAH

The promise of Matrix Healing is ultimately much larger than
that of being able to heal ourselves, though we have that

promise, too. In the end, however, our goal is to heal not only ourselves but also our entire world; indeed, if we truly understand Matrix Healing, we begin to see that they are inseparable. For in order to truly heal ourselves, we must desire to heal all who suffer and to remove darkness wherever it is found.

As always, I turn to the words of the Zohar, which eloquently describe this process of awakening to this higher calling: "I was asleep but my heart was awakened. . . . It is the voice of my beloved that knocks, saying, 'Open to Me, my sister. . . . Open to Me an opening no bigger than the eye of a needle, and I will open to thee the Supernal Gates. Open to Me, my sister, because thou art the door through which there is an entrance to Me. If thou open'st not, I am closed.'"

When I first became acquainted with the Bible codes I mentioned in the Introduction, I was struck by the dire prophecies that they apparently contained. Frequently, worldwide catastrophes were mentioned, some with details that seemed shockingly contemporary—and, accordingly, quite frightening.

Yet beside each possible catastrophe appeared the words *Will you change this?* Clearly, we humans have the power to avert the ecological and political catastrophes that threaten not only our individual health but also the survival of our entire planet. We have the power to end the new epidemics of so many diseases and to end pain and suffering. Today, as the 2,000-year-old Kabbalah finally becomes available to us, as we have finally learned to crack the Bible codes, as we truly understand that we live in a global village, we have the opportunity—and the responsibility—to revitalize and respiritualize our world, to recapture the soulfulness in the world to which we have been blind—until now.

So in response to that question within the Torah, my answer is a resounding Yes! *Together we will change this,* so that we can finally see the end of suffering. Together we can bring about the prophecy in the Essene Book of Revelations: "And I saw a new heaven and a new earth. I heard a voice saying there shall be no more death, neither sorrow nor crying, for the former things are passed away."

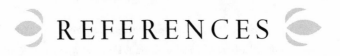

REFERENCES

FOREWORD

Dossey, L. *Healing Words.* San Francisco: HarperSanFrancisco, 1993.

_____. *Reinventing Medicine.* San Francisco: HarperSanFrancisco, 1999.

Koenig, H. G., M. E. McCullough, and D. B. Larson. *Handbook of Religion and Health.* New York: Oxford University Press, 2000.

Underhill, E. *Practical Mysticism.* New York: Dutton, 1915.

Webster's New Twentieth Century Dictionary, unabridged 2nd ed. New York: World, 1971.

INTRODUCTION

Satinover, Jeffrey, M.D. *Cracking the Bible Code.* New York: William Morrow, 1977.

Wolf, Fred Alan. *Parallel Universes: The Search for Other Worlds.* New York: Simon & Schuster, 1990.

CHAPTER 1

Alison, T. G., et al. "Medical and Economic Costs of Psychological Distress in Patients with Coronary Artery Disease." *Mayo Clinic Proceedings* 70, no. 8 (1995): 743–52.

Browne, Malcolm W. "Quantum Theory: Disturbing Questions Remain Unresolved." *New York Times,* February 11, 1986, C3.

Einstein, Albert. *Ideas and Opinions.* New York: Bonanza Books, 1988.

Jahn, Robert G., and Brenda J. Dunne. *Margins of Reality: The Role of Consciousness in the Physical World.* New York: Harcourt Brace Jovanovich, 1987.

Kreiter, Marcella S. "Generous Oldsters Live Longer." United Press International, November 13, 2002.

McDonald, A. B. "Ups and Downs of Neutrino Oscillation." *Science News* 117, no. 24 (June 14, 1980): 377–83.

Minkler, Meredith. "People Need People: Social Support and Health." Chapter 8 in Robert Ornstein and Charles Swencroinis, eds., *The Healing Brain: A Scientific Reader.* Cambridge, MA: Malor Books, 1999.

Penninx, B., et al. "Effects of Social Support and Personal Coping Resources on Mortality and Older Age: Longitudinal Aging Study (Amsterdam)." *American Journal of Epidemiology* 146, no. 6 (1997): 510–19.

Pontecorvo, Bruno. "Soviet Neutrinos Have Mass." *New Scientist* 105, no. 1446 (March 7, 1985): 23.

Schwartz, Jeffrey M., and Sharon Begley. *The Mind and the Brain: Neuroplasticity and the Power of Mental Force.* New York: Regan Books, 2002.

Sutton, Christine. "The Secret Life of the Neutrino." *New Scientist* 117, no. 1585 (January 14, 1988): 53–57.

Talbot, Michael. *The Holographic Universe.* New York: Harper Perennial, 1991.

Thomsen, Dietrick E. "Anomalons Get More and More Anomalous." *Science News* 125 (February 25, 1984), pp 17–19.

Langer, E. J., and J. Rodin. "The Effects of Choice and Enhanced Personal Responsibility for the Aged: A Field Experiment in an Institutional Setting." *Journal of Personality and Social Psychology* 34 (1916): 191–198.

CHAPTER 2

Berg, Yehuda. *The Power of Kabbalah.* San Diego: Jodere, 2001.

Chase, Truddi. *When Rabbit Howls.* New York: Dutton, 1987.

Goleman, Daniel. "New Focus on Multiple Personality." *New York Times,* May 21, 1985, C1.

———. "Probing the Enigma of Multiple Personality." *New York Times,* June 25, 1988, C1.

Hurley, Thomas J., III. "Inner Faces of Multiplicity." *Investigations* 1, no. 3/4 (1985): 4.

Talbot, Michael. *The Holographic Universe.* New York: Harper Perennial, 1991.

CHAPTER 3

Baudelaire, Charles P. *On Wine and Hashish,* trans. Andrew Brown. Albany, NY: Hesperus Press, 2003.

Matt, Daniel Chanan. *The Essential Kabbalah: The Heart of Jewish Mysticism.* Edison, NJ: Castle Books, 1997.

Wolf, Rabbi Laibl. *Practical Kabbalah: A Guide to Jewish Wisdom for Everyday Life.* New York: Three Rivers Press, 1999.

CHAPTER 4

De Charmes, R. "Personal Causation: The Internal Affective Determinants of Behavior." New York: Academic Press (1968).

Pollard, Jeffrey W., et al. "Revolution in Evolution." *Einstein Journal* (Fall 1991).

Rein, Glen, and Rollin McCraty. "Modulation of DNA by Coherent Heart Frequencies." *Proceedings of the 3rd Annual Conference of the ISSEEM,* Monterey, CA, June 1993: 2.

Schwartz, Jeffrey M., and Sharon Begley. *The Mind and the Brain: Neuroplasticity and the Power of Mental Force.* New York: Regan Books, 2002.

CHAPTER 5

Cousens, Gabriel, M.D. *Conscious Eating.* Berkeley, CA: North Atlantic Books, 2000.

The Essene Gospel of Peace, Book One. International Biogenic Society. British Columbian Canada: International Biogenic Society, 1981.

Kazantzakis, Nikos. *Zorba the Greek.* New York: Simon & Schuster, 1952.

Kellman, Raphael. *Gut Reactions.* New York: Broadway Books, 2002.

CHAPTER 6

Batmanghelidj, Fereydoon, M.D. *Your Body's Many Cries for Water.* Vermont: Global Health Solutions, 1997.

Ryrie, Charles. *The Healing Power of Water.* Boston: Journey Editions, 1999.

CHAPTER 7

Cantin, M., and J. Genest. "The Heart As an Endocrine Gland." *Scientific American* 254 (1986): 76.

Childre, Doc Lew. *Cut-Thru: Achieve Total Security and Maximum Energy.* Boulder Creek, CA: Planetary Publications, 1995.

Frasure-Smith, N., F. Lesperance, and M. Talasic. "Depression Following Myocardial Infarction: Impact on 6-Month Survival." *JAMA* 270, no. 15 (1993): 1860–61.

Goodman, M., G. Moran, H. Meilman, J. Quigley, and M. Sherman. "Hostility predicts restenosis after percutaneous transluminal coronary angioplasty." Mayo Clinic Proceedings 71 (1996): 729–734

Hafen, B., et al. *The Health Effects of Attitudes Emotions and Relationships.* Provo, UT: EMS Associates, 1992.

Hall, H., L. Minnes, and K. Olness. "The Psychophysiology of Voluntary Immunomodulation." *International Journal of Neuroscience* 69 (1993): 221–34.

Kaplan, George A., et al. "Depression Amplifies the Association Between Carotid Atherosclerosis and LDL, Fibrinogen, and Smoking." Report at the 1992 American Heart Association Annual Meeting on Cardiovascular Epidemiology, Cleveland, Ohio.

Kaplan, R. "The Role of Nature in the Context of the Workplace." *Landscape and Urban Planning* 26 (1993): 193–201.

Kawachi, J., et al. "Symptoms of Anxiety and Risk of Coronary Heart Disease: The Normative Aging Study." *Circulation* 90 (1994): 2225–9.

Luks, Allan. *The Healing Power of Doing Good: The Health and Spiritual Benefits of Helping Others.* New York: Ballantine, 1991.

McClelland, D., and C. Kirshnit. "The Effect of Motivational Arousal Through Films on Salivary Immunoglobulin A." *Psychology and Health* 2 (1987): 31–52.

Ornstein, Robert, and David Sobel. "Can We Voluntarily Alter Immune Function?" *Mental Med Update* 11, no. 2 (1993).

_____. *The Healing Brain.* Cambridge, MA: Makor Books, 1987.

Pearsall, Paul. *The Heart's Code.* New York: Broadway Books, 1998.

Rein, G., R. M. McCraty, and M. Atkinson. "Effects of Positive and Negative Emotions on Salivary IgA." *Journal for the Advancement of Medicine* 8, no. 2 (1995): 87–105.

Sapse, A. T. "Type A Behavior and Elevated Psychological and Neurological Responses to Cognitive Tasks." *Science* 218 (1982): 483–85.

Schwartz, Jeffrey M., and Sharon Begley. *The Mind and the Brain: Neuroplasticity and the Power of Mental Force.* New York: Regan Books, 2002.

Ulrich, R. S. "View Through a Window May Influence Recovery from Surgery." *Science* 224 (1984): 420–21.

Williams, R. *Anger Kills: Seventeen Strategies for Controlling the Anger That Can Harm Your Health.* New York: Times Books, 1993.

_____. *The Trusting Heart.* New York: Times Books, 1989.

CHAPTER 8

Berg, Yehuda. *The 72 Names of God: Technology for the Soul.* New York: Kabbalah Publishing, 2003.

Schwartz, Jeffrey M., and Sharon Begley. *The Mind and the Brain: Neuroplasticity and the Power of Mental Force.* New York: Regan Books, 2002.

Speigel, D., et al. "The Effect of Psychosocial Treatment on Survival of Patients with Metastatic Breast Cancer." *Lancet* 11 (1989): 888–91.

Targ, Elisabeth. *Reinventing Medicine.* San Francisco: HarperSanFrancisco, 1999.

CHAPTER 9

Cohen, Mark, and Rabbi Yehuda Lev Ashlag, "In the Shadow of the Ladder." In Rabbi Bergh Ashlag, *In the Shadow of the Ladder,* trans. Mark Cohen and Yedidah Cohen. Safed, Israel: Nehora Press, 2002.

Dossey, Larry, M.D. *Meaning and Medicine: Lessons from a Doctor's Tales of Breakthrough and Healing.* New York: Bantam Books, 1991.

Levin, Jeff, M.D. *God, Faith, and Health: Exploring the Spirituality-Healing Connection.* New York: John Wiley, 2002.

Manocha, K. *Dialogues with Scientists and Sages.* New York: Routledge & Kegan Paul, 1986.

Neal, H. *The Politics of Pain.* New York: McGraw-Hill, 1977.

Weber, Renee. "Philosophical Foundations and Frameworks for Healing." *ReVision* 2, no. 2 (1979): 66–77.

CHAPTER 10

Abulafia, Abraham. Sefer Ha Yasher, trans. Moshe Idel. *Studies in Ecstatic Kabbalah.* New York: State University of New York, 1988.

Cooper, David A., Rabbi. *God Is a Verb.* New York: Penguin, 1998.

ACKNOWLEDGMENTS

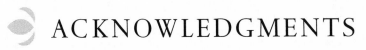

PSALM 111—

The beginning of wisdom is the awe of God.

WE do not conceive of new ideas, and we ourselves do not discover new facts and theories. Rather, they flow through us, they are a gift, they are a reflection of the beneficence of God.

Many people helped bring this book to fruition, and I am deeply appreciative of all their hard work. First and foremost, many thanks to Rachel Kranz, who helped make this book a reality. Her unique ability to translate ethereal ideas into simple and clear language was a gift for me. Her ideas always seem to challenge and encourage me at the same time. Special thanks to my editor, Kim Meisner. Her enthusiasm, intelligence, and warmth helped make this project so special.

Special thanks to Kitty Farmer, who is one of my great supporters and is relentless in her desire to get life transforming ideas out to others. Special thanks to Larry Dossey, M.D., who has been an inspiration for me for so many years. Connecting with kindred souls is living life deeply.

Thanks to the following people, who helped in a variety of ways: Barry Kellman, Mara Goodman, Grace Ruiz, Eric Staff.

INDEX

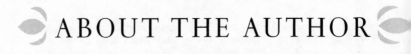

ABOUT THE AUTHOR

RAPHAEL KELLMAN, M.D., an internist by training, graduated from the Albert Einstein College of Medicine in 1987. He has been studying Kabbalah for many years and has long searched for the healing messages in ancient mystical tradition. He studies Kabbalah with some of the greatest kabbalists in Israel.

He is known for his unique and seamless integration of the spiritual, psychological, ecological, and physical dimensions to healing into not only a new unified and soulful medicine, but an enchanted view of life as well.

He is the founder and medical director of the Kellman Center for Progressive Medicine, and the author of *Gut Reactions*.